Contemporary Cardiovascular Continuum™

Ezra A. Amsterdam, MD
Professor of Medicine
Director, Cardiac Care Unit, Division of Cardiovascular Medicine
University of California, Davis, School of Medicine
Sacramento, California

Denise D. Barnard, MD
Associate Professor of Medicine
Associate Director, Heart Failure/Cardiac Transplantation Program
University of California, San Diego

Barry H. Greenberg, MD
Professor of Medicine
Director, Heart Failure/Cardiac Transplantation Program
University of California, San Diego

Scott M. Grundy, MD, PhD
Director, Center for Human Nutrition,
and Chairman, Department of Clinical Nutrition,
University of Texas Southwestern Medical Center, Dallas

Philip R. Liebson, MD
Professor of Medicine
McMullay-Eykel Chair in Cardiology
Associate Director, Section of Cardiology, Rush Medical College
Rush-Presbyterian-St. Luke's Medical Center, Chicago, Illinois

Published by Handbooks in Health Care Co.,
Newtown, Pennsylvania, USA

This book has been prepared and is presented as a service to the medical community. The information provided reflects the knowledge, experience, and personal opinions of Ezra A. Amsterdam, MD, Professor of Medicine, Director, Cardiac Care Unit, Division of Cardiovascular Medicine, University of California, Davis, School of Medicine, Sacramento, California; Denise D. Barnard, MD, Associate Professor of Medicine, Associate Director, Heart Failure/Cardiac Transplantation Program, University of California, San Diego, CA; Barry H. Greenberg, MD, Professor of Medicine, Director, Heart Failure/Cardiac Transplantation Program, University of California, San Diego, CA; Scott M. Grundy, MD, PhD, Director, Center for Human Nutrition, Chairman, Department of Clinical Nutrition, University of Texas Southwestern Medical Center, Dallas; and Philip R. Liebson, MD, Professor of Medicine, McMullay-Eykel Chair in Cardiology, Associate Director, Section of Cardiology, Rush Medical College, Rush-Presbyterian-St. Luke's Medical Center, Chicago, Illinois.

This book is not intended to replace or to be used as a substitute for the complete prescribing information prepared by each manufacturer for each drug. Because of possible variations in drug indications, in dosage information, in newly described toxicities, in drug/drug interactions, and in other items of importance, reference to such complete prescribing information is definitely recommended before any of the drugs discussed are used or prescribed.

International Standard Book Number: 1-931981-71-X

Library of Congress Catalog Card Number: 2006935389

CONTENTS

Foreword

The understanding that cardiovascular diseases are not discontinuous, self-contained events but rather points on a continuum that extends from 'normality' to end-stage heart failure has been an important conceptual advance that has strongly influenced our approach to treating patients. This continuum defines a cycle that is initiated by the presence of a constellation of cardiovascular risk factors in otherwise 'healthy' asymptomatic patients. Over time, these risk factors result in structural abnormalities in the heart. These abnormalities can be due either insidiously to the long-standing effects of hypertension and diabetes, or more abruptly with an acute myocardial infarction (MI). In either case, further remodeling of the heart leads to progressive deterioration in cardiac function and the development of heart failure, a condition that is associated with substantial morbidity and mortality. In noting these associations and their implications, health-care practitioners can better serve patients by treating manifest disease and by preventing disease from occurring (primary prevention) or progressing (secondary prevention). This text presents a comprehensive overview of the continuum of cardiovascular disease that extends from the presence of risk factors to cardiac damage to the development of heart failure and its subsequent sequelae.

This very concept has been formalized in the *American College of Cardiology/American Heart Association 2005 Guideline for the diagnosis and management of heart failure in the adult,* which groups patients into four stages according to the severity of their condition. A patient at risk for developing heart failure is considered to be Stage A, while a patient with structural damage to the heart who has not yet developed the well-recognized signs and symptoms of heart failure is designated as Stage B. A patient with symptomatic heart failure is considered to be Stage C, and an end-stage patient with refractory heart failure is defined as Stage D. This staging system also emphasizes that *early* treatment is essentially the *best* treatment. It implies that the practitioner should consider what potentially lies ahead for the patient when initiating therapies. Thus, a high-risk cardiovascular patient with the metabolic syndrome should receive treatments designed to reduce the level of risk factors and to prevent the future likelihood of myocardial damage. A post-MI patient should receive treatment that both reduces the reinfarction rate and prevents maladaptive structural remodeling that results in heart failure. If heart failure occurs, therapy should be designed to relieve signs and symptoms and prevent further progression to end-stage disease.

Over the years, our understanding of basic pathophysiologic mechanisms responsible for the cardiovascular diseases described in this text has grown exponentially. Interestingly, there are common threads throughout the cardiovascular continuum, including the presence of an inflammatory component, the adverse effects of sustained neurohormonal activation, and the maladaptive nature of many compensatory mechanisms that come into play in response to cardiac stress or damage. One of the most important advances in therapy has been to direct specific therapies toward correcting or at least attenuating these underlying abnormalities wherever possible.

The authors hope that the information presented here will help the practitioner better recognize the connections between the high-risk patient with the metabolic syndrome, the patient who has suffered an MI, and the patient who is being treated for heart failure. Most importantly, knowledge of the continuum of cardiovascular disease should lead to the use of more appropriate therapies and their initiation in a more timely manner.

Barry H. Greenberg, MD
Professor of Medicine
Director, Heart Failure/Cardiac Transplantation Program
University of California, San Diego

Chapter **1**

The Metabolic Syndrome as a Multiplex Risk Factor

The metabolic syndrome consists of a clustering of risk factors for atherosclerotic cardiovascular disease (ASCVD).[1] These risk factors include atherogenic dyslipidemia, elevated blood pressure, elevated plasma glucose, a prothrombotic state, and a proinflammatory state. Nearly 25% of the adult population in the United States is now estimated to have the metabolic syndrome.[2] Although ASCVD must be considered the most important clinical end point in the United States, the association between the metabolic syndrome and type 2 diabetes is strong,[3] and even prominent in many countries. Type 2 diabetes itself is strongly associated with ASCVD.

Pathogenesis of the Metabolic Syndrome

The two dominant underlying risk factors of the metabolic syndrome are obesity and insulin resistance.[3] Large amounts of adipose tissue in obese people is increasingly being recognized as the producer of factors that contribute to the development of the metabolic syndrome. These factors include excess nonesterified fatty acids, cytokines (tumor necrosis factor-α [TNF-α]), resistin, adiponectin, leptin, and plasminogen activator inhibitor-1 (PAI-1). A notable feature of the metabolic syndrome is accumulation of fat in tissue outside of adipose tissue, notably, muscle and liver. This ectopic deposition of fat appears to play an important role in development of metabolic risk

7

factors. Beyond obesity, other abnormalities of adipose tissue are associated with the metabolic syndrome, including abdominal obesity[4] and lipodystrophy.[5]

Most people with the metabolic syndrome display some degree of insulin resistance, which many investigators[6,7] regard as a critical link in the pathogenesis of the metabolic syndrome. Clearly, insulin resistance is a major underlying risk factor for type 2 diabetes. Although insulin resistance is strongly associated with other metabolic risk factors for ASCVD, evidence that it is a direct cause is less clear. Various plausible mechanisms have been proposed to explain how insulin resistance could induce these risk factors.[6,7] Perhaps the best opportunity for understanding the relationship between insulin resistance and metabolic risk factors lies in further study of cases of primary (genetic) insulin resistance.[8] Preliminary evidence suggests that genetic forms of insulin resistance may produce mild aberrations in metabolic risk factors independent of obesity. Moreover, in some people, obesity and primary insulin resistance may together exacerbate these risk factors.

Other underlying risk factors for the metabolic syndrome include physical inactivity, aging, atherogenic diets, and hormonal imbalance.[3] Physical inactivity worsens insulin resistance and promotes development of obesity. Loss of muscle mass and increase in body fat commonly accompany aging. Aging muscle further exhibits some loss in ability to oxidize fatty acids, which will increase insulin resistance. Postulated endocrine abnormalities underlying the metabolic syndrome include polycystic ovary disease and mild hypercorticoidism.

Genetic heterogeneity affects expression of individual metabolic risk components, ie, lipoprotein metabolism, blood pressure levels, insulin secretory capacity, coagulation and fibrinolysis factors, and inflammatory responses. In other words, the genetic architecture for each of these systems falls under the influence of the underlying risk factors.

Risk Assessment in Patients With the Metabolic Syndrome

A commonly asked question is whether the metabolic syndrome itself can be used to assess the likelihood of developing ASCVD. Prospective studies[9] have shown that individuals with the metabolic syndrome are at increased risk for ASCVD. Recently, investigators of the Framingham Heart Study carried out an analysis to determine the absolute risk for ASCVD associated with the metabolic syndrome.[3] It seems evident that a condition characterized by multiple risk factors will carry a greater risk for adverse clinical outcomes than will a single risk factor. This conclusion is implicit in Framingham risk equations, which incorporate many of the components of the metabolic syndrome. The Framingham analysis was based on Framingham study offspring (men and women, mean age 52 years) who were followed for 8 years. The investigators found that the metabolic syndrome alone predicted approximately 25% of all new-onset ASCVD. This percentage was largely unaffected by whether diabetes was included in the metabolic syndrome criteria. In the absence of diabetes, people with the metabolic syndrome rarely exhibited a 10-year risk for coronary heart disease (CHD) exceeding 20%, which is designated high-risk by the Third Report of the Expert Panel on Detection, Evaluation, and Treatment in Adults (Adult Treatment Panel III [ATP III]). Most men with the metabolic syndrome had a 10-year risk of 10% to 20%, which ATP III calls moderately high risk. Framingham women with the metabolic syndrome usually had lower risk (ie, a 10-year risk for major coronary events less than 10%). Importantly, Framingham investigators showed that a diagnosis of the metabolic syndrome provides a less-accurate assessment of 10-year risk than does the Framingham risk scoring procedure that makes use of all of the major risk factors. Thus, the metabolic syndrome per se should not be used for global risk assessment. Instead, standard risk algorithms are preferred for this purpose.[1]

The Metabolic Syndrome as a Predictor of Diabetes

According to Framingham investigators, the metabolic syndrome is highly predictive of new-onset diabetes.[3] The relative risk for developing type 2 diabetes is approximately five-fold higher in people with the metabolic syndrome than in those without it. The predictive power for diabetes may be enhanced by carrying out an oral glucose tolerance test. An oral glucose tolerance test (OGTT) may identify patients who are normoglycemic but have impaired glucose tolerance. These patients will likely be at higher risk for developing type 2 diabetes than those who remain glucose tolerant.

Management of Underlying Risk Factors

First-line therapy of the metabolic syndrome is to modify the underlying risk factors: overweight and obesity, physical inactivity, and an atherogenic diet. Clinical management represents an extension of the public health approach to risk reduction. When a person is identified by ATP III criteria to have the metabolic syndrome, he or she should enter clinical management. The physician should set the goals of treatment, encourage lifestyle modification, and involve additional health professionals as necessary.

Overweight and Obesity

Overweight and obesity contribute significantly to raising blood pressure levels in many populations. For almost any population or subgroup, levels of blood pressure on average are higher in overweight/obese people than in lean individuals. The mechanisms underlying this association are not well understood, but several factors have been implicated. These include increases in peripheral vascular resistance and increases in blood volume leading to a higher cardiac output. Of the several implicated factors, an increased reabsorption of sodium is highly suspect.[10] Enhanced sodium reabsorption has been attributed to an elevated glomerular filtration rate as well as to increased renal blood flow.[11] Hall et al further speculate that altered intrarenal physical forces secondary to kidney compression by excess adipose tissue are yet another factor increasing sodium reabsorption. This and other mechanisms may be responsible for activation of the renin-angiotensin system, which in turn may impair natriuresis.[12] Increased angiotensin will raise peripheral resistance even further. Moreover, obese people appear to have an overactive sympathetic nervous system, which will increase cardiac output and raise peripheral resistance. Overproduction of leptin accompanying obesity may raise blood pressure further, possibly through interaction of leptin with other neurochemical pathways in the hypothalamus, including melanocortin-4 receptors.[13] Many of these pathways are at present conjectural, but continue to be foci of ongoing research.

Treatment of obesity should follow the guidelines developed by the National Institutes of Health in 1998.[14] According to these guidelines, overweight and obesity are defined as body mass indexes (BMIs) of 25 to 29.9 kg/m^2 and ≥30 kg/m^2, respectively. Abdominal obesity was added to the classification and was defined as a waist circumference ≥102 cm (≥40 inches) in men and ≥88 cm (≥35 inches) in women. Abdominal obesity appears to be strongly associated with the metabolic risk factors for ASCVD.[14] ATP III recommends that abdominal obesity be one of the clinical criteria for diagnosis of the metabolic syndrome. However, some people will manifest the metabolic syndrome at waist circumferences less than the categoric cut points listed in the obesity guidelines.

Weight reduction in obese people will help to reverse most of the metabolic risk factors.[14] The essential approach to weight reduction involves behavior changes to reduce caloric intake and increase physical activity. Treatment guidelines emphasize certain key points. For example, 'crash diets' and 'extreme diets' rarely achieve long-term weight reduction. More effective for long-term weight loss is moderate reduction in caloric intake that eliminates about

500 to 1,000 calories a day. A realistic goal for weight reduction is 7% to 10% during the first 6 to 12 months. To achieve long-term weight loss, addition of regular physical activity is usually required. A key point for long-term success is the need for behavior modification. Dieting alone is rarely successful. Behavior modification includes an improvement in eating habits. Among the habits that typically cause weight gain are a failure to plan meals ahead of time, failure to choose lower-calorie foods (eg, failure to read labels), snacking between meals and at bedtime, overeating at meals (eg, large portions, second helpings, desserts), frequent dining out, and being prone to eating binges. Useful techniques of behavior modification include family support, managing and preventing periods of stress, and daily exercise. For motivated patients, the obesity guidelines for weight reduction can be obtained online at www.nhlbi.nih.gov and www.americanheart.org. An understanding of principles of behavior modification is important but frequently insufficient. For many patients in clinical management, professional support (eg, nutritional counseling) can assist in achieving weight reduction.

Physical Inactivity

Most American adults are sedentary. This is unfortunate because regular physical activity promotes weight reduction, reduces insulin resistance, mitigates metabolic risk factors, and reduces risk for several chronic diseases. Among the latter are ASCVD and type 2 diabetes. Physical inactivity is an underlying risk factor for the metabolic syndrome. The American Heart Association (AHA) provides physical activity guidelines that are moderate and practical.[15] The basic recommendation is a daily minimum of 30 minutes of moderate-intensity physical activity. Some additional benefit is achieved by increasing exercise time to 1 hour a day. Suggestions that may promote increased physical activity include:[16]

- Walking briskly (10 to 15 minutes) several times per day
- Adding exercise to daily habits (brisk walking, jogging, swimming, biking, golfing, team sports)

- Substituting exercise activities for television viewing and computer games
- Purchasing simple exercise equipment for the home (eg, treadmill).

Dietary Modification

The concept that dietary factors independent of obesity elevate blood pressure has evoked interest in the public health community. Considerable epidemiologic and clinical research has been carried out to test this hypothesis. Several dietary components have been put forward as potential factors in the development of hypertension. These include high intakes of sodium, calcium, and fat, as well as low intakes of potassium, fruits, and vegetables. Considerable data support the concept that some individuals are 'salt sensitive' and undergo a rise in blood pressure with high-salt diets. Up to one third of the population is believed to be susceptible to salt-induced hypertension.

The relationship between high calcium intake and hypertension is less well established. The likelihood that dietary factors are important in the etiology of hypertension has led to experimentation with diets designed to improve nutrient composition as it relates to blood pressure. One widely tested diet is the Dietary Approaches to Stop Hypertension (DASH) diet,[17] which is low in fat and high in fruits, vegetables, and fiber, and tends to be low in sodium and high in potassium. Rigid adherence to the DASH diet causes a moderate reduction in blood pressure in hypertensive patients.

The Dietary Guidelines for Americans, set forth by the US Departments of Agriculture and Health and Human Services, offer a reasonable dietary approach for managing patients with the metabolic syndrome.[18] The key features of dietary recommendations based on these guidelines and those of the ATP III panel are listed in Table 1-1.

The AHA (www.americanheart.org) provides useful information on how to choose a healthy eating pattern that will reduce risk for ASCVD in patients with the metabolic syndrome.

Table 1-1: Key Features of Dietary Recommendations

- Choose a variety of fruits and vegetables daily

- Avoid excess dietary saturated fat
  - Choose a diet that is low in saturated fat and cholesterol and moderate in total fat
  - Replace saturated fats with unsaturated oils

- Avoid excess dietary carbohydrates
  - For carbohydrates, emphasize grain foods, especially whole grains
  - Choose beverages and foods to moderate intake of sugars

- Choose and prepare foods with less salt

- If you drink alcoholic beverages, do so in moderation

Modified from Dietary Guidelines for Americans, US Departments of Agriculture and Health and Human Services, 2000.

Management of Individual Metabolic Risk Factors

Atherogenic Dyslipidemia

In patients with the metabolic syndrome who have atherogenic dyslipidemia, the primary target of therapy is elevated apo B-containing lipoproteins. The best indicators for these lipoproteins are low-density lipoproteins (LDL) plus very low-density lipoprotein cholesterol (VLDL-C) (non-high-density lipoprotein cholesterol [non-HDL-C]) or total apo B.[1] For high-risk patients (10-year risk for major coronary events >20%), the goal of therapy is to reduce non-HDL-C to <130 mg/dL (or apo B to <90 mg/dL). For those at moderately high risk (10-year risk

10% to 20%), the goal of therapy is non-HDL-C <160 mg/dL (or apo B <110 mg/dL). For both categories of risk, statin therapy usually is indicated. Statins reduce both LDL-apo B and VLDL-apo B. In many patients, the goal can be achieved with statin therapy alone.

If triglyceride levels remain elevated after statin therapy in patients at high or moderately high risk, physicians should consider adding a fibrate or nicotinic acid.[1] The preferred fibrate to use in combination with a statin is fenofibrate (TriCor®, Lofibra™) because the combination of a statin and gemfibrozil (Lopid®) carries too high a risk for severe myopathy. Available data indicate that the combination of a statin and fenofibrate carries a lower risk for myopathy. When fenofibrate is used in combination with a statin, there often is some additional lowering of total apo B (or non-HDL-C), but the combination offers three advantages. First, fenofibrate reduces atherogenic remnant lipoproteins; second, it transforms smaller LDL to larger LDL; and third, it raises HDL-C more than statins alone.[19] The same benefits are achieved by combining a statin with nicotinic acid. Unfortunately, nicotinic acid often causes bothersome side effects, including flushing and itching of the skin, gastrointestinal distress, rises in plasma glucose and uric acid, and abnormal liver function tests. Both flushing and abnormal liver function tests can be minimized by use of an extended-release niacin preparation (Niaspan®). Long-acting preparations carry too high a risk for liver dysfunction, while crystalline nicotinic acid more often causes severe flushing. When nicotinic acid is used with statin therapy, the dose should be kept relatively low (1 to 2 g/d).

When patients with the metabolic syndrome and atherogenic dyslipidemia have a 10-year risk <10% (lower to moderate risk), drug therapy should be used only when the non-HDL-C (or apo B) is high (ie, non-HDL-C >190 mg/dL or apo B >130 mg/dL). Otherwise, lifestyle therapies should be emphasized.

Elevated Blood Pressure

The Seventh Report of the Joint National Committee on Prevention, Detection, Evaluation, and Treatment of High Blood Pressure (JNC 7)[20] recommends the use of antihypertensive drugs when blood pressure exceeds 140 mm Hg systolic or 90 mm Hg diastolic on repeated measurements. The primary goal of therapy is to reduce blood pressure to <140/90 mm Hg. In patients with established diabetes, JNC 7 sets a lower goal, <130/80 mm Hg. JNC 7 did not identify particular antihypertensive agents as preferable for hypertensive patients with the metabolic syndrome. However, thiazide diuretics and β-blockers in high doses can accentuate insulin resistance and worsen atherogenic dyslipidemia. In the metabolic syndrome, higher doses of thiazides can cause an elevation of glucose to categoric diabetes in patients with impaired glucose tolerance. Therefore, doses of thiazide diuretics should be relatively low. Despite a worsening of glucose tolerance, β-blockers protect against sudden death in patients with established ASCVD; consequently, they are not contraindicated in patients with type 2 diabetes and ASCVD. Angiotensin-converting enzyme (ACE) inhibitors and angiotensin-receptor blockers (ARBs) are especially attractive for patients with the metabolic syndrome because they are renoprotective and have been shown to reduce risk for new-onset ASCVD. Several clinical trials, but not all, point to advantages of ACE inhibitors and ARBs over other drugs in patients with diabetes.[20]

Insulin Resistance and Hyperglycemia

Much interest has focused on the possibility that insulin resistance raises blood pressure. Several studies demonstrate that people with hypertension are insulin resistant.[13, 21] This fact undoubtedly engendered the concept of a cause-and-effect relationship (ie, insulin resistance causes hypertension). With this focus, it follows that obesity contributes to higher blood pressure through insulin resistance.

Several of the pathways to hypertension once attributed to obesity likewise have been attributed to insulin resistance. Despite interest in the role of insulin resistance in blood pressure elevation, the mechanistic relationship remains undetermined. Moreover, epidemiologic studies indicate that certain populations carrying a high burden of insulin resistance, such as South Asians and Native Americans, are not particularly prone to hypertension. In other words, in the presence of isolated primary insulin resistance, the frequency of hypertension does not appear to be increased. For this reason, insulin resistance per se may not be a major cause of hypertension. This contrasts to the almost certain role of obesity as a cause of high blood pressure, whatever the mechanisms.

A fundamental question is whether drug treatment of insulin resistance will reduce the risk for developing type 2 diabetes and, if so, whether it is cost-effective. Evidence is growing that drugs can reduce risk for conversion of impaired glucose tolerance into categoric hyperglycemia (or diabetes). Metformin (Glucophage®) therapy in patients with prediabetes reduced the risk for conversion to diabetes.[22]

Insulin resistance is associated with increased ASCVD risk. In one clinical trial, metformin therapy appeared to decrease the risk for new-onset ASCVD in an obese subgroup.[23] Further studies with metformin are required to document a cardioprotective effect. None of the glitazones (thiazolidinediones) have been documented to reduce risk for ASCVD, although in one clinical trial, suggestive evidence of benefit was obtained.[24]

These considerations lead to the issue of how best to treat insulin resistance and hyperglycemia in patients with type 2 diabetes. When hyperglycemia develops in patients with the metabolic syndrome, the risk for ASCVD rises. In patients with type 2 diabetes, priority must be given to appropriate treatment of dyslipidemia and hypertension. Drug therapy of each has been documented to reduce risk for ASCVD.[1,20] A strong case can be made for improved glycemic control as well. Most importantly, good glycemic control will reduce risk for microvascular disease and other diabetic complications. For these reasons, a reduction in glycated hemoglobin (Hb A_{1c}) level to <7.0% is indicated. Whether better control will reduce ASCVD events remains to be documented in controlled clinical trials, although circumstantial evidence strongly suggests that it will.

Prothrombotic State

The various prothrombotic factors typical of the metabolic syndrome, including elevations of fibrinogen and PAI-1, are not routinely measured in clinical practice. Nonetheless, in both primary and secondary prevention, thrombotic events can be reduced by aspirin therapy. The AHA has recommended use of low-dose aspirin (81 mg/d) for most patients whose 10-year risk for CHD is >10%, as determined by Framingham risk scoring.[25] When patients with the metabolic syndrome have a 10-year risk for major coronary events >10%, aspirin prophylaxis should be considered.

Proinflammatory State

This condition is best recognized by elevations of C-reactive protein (CRP), but various inflammatory cytokines (eg, TNF-α, IL-6) and fibrinogen are commonly elevated as well. Patients with the metabolic syndrome typically have elevations in CRP levels (eg, >3 mg/dL).[26] There is no specific therapy for high levels of CRP. Nonetheless, weight reduction and many of the drugs used to treat metabolic risk factors will lower CRP. This change could represent a dampening of the proinflammatory state.

References

1. Third Report of the National Cholesterol Education Program (NCEP) Expert Panel on Detection, Evaluation, and Treatment of High Blood Cholesterol in Adults (Adult Treatment Panel III) final report. *Circulation* 2002;106:3143-3421.

2. Ford ES, Giles WH, Dietz WH: Prevalence of the metabolic syndrome among US adults: findings from the third National Health and Nutrition Survey. *JAMA* 2002;287:356-359.

3. Grundy SM, Brewer HB Jr, Cleeman JI, et al: Definition of metabolic syndrome: report of the National Heart, Lung, and Blood Institute/American Heart Association conference on scientific issues related to definition. *Circulation* 2004;109:433-438.

4. Frayn KN: Visceral fat and insulin resistance—causative or correlative? *Br J Nutr* 2000;83(suppl 1):S71-S77.

5. Garg A: Acquired and inherited lipodystrophies. *N Engl J Med* 2004;350:1220-1234.

6. Reaven GM: Banting lecture 1988. Role of insulin resistance in human disease. *Diabetes* 1988;37:1595-1607.

7. Ferrannini E, Haffner SM, Mitchell BD: Hyperinsulinemia: the key feature of a cardiovascular and metabolic syndrome. *Diabetologia* 1991;34:416-422.

8. Abate N, Carulli L, Cabo-Chan A Jr, et al: Genetic polymorphism PC-1 K121Q and ethnic susceptibility to insulin resistance. *Clin Endocrinol Metab* 2003;88:5927-5934.

9. Lakka HM, Laaksonen DE, Lakka TA, et al: The metabolic syndrome and total and cardiovascular disease mortality in middle-aged men. *JAMA* 2002;288:2709-2716.

10. Hall JE: The kidney, hypertension, and obesity. *Hypertension* 2003;41:625-633.

11. Hall JE: Mechanisms of abnormal renal sodium handling in obesity hypertension. *Am J Hypertens* 1997;10:49S-55S.

12. Hall JE, Hildebrandt DA, Kuo J: Obesity hypertension: role of leptin and sympathetic nervous system. *Am J Hypertens* 2001; 14:103S-115S.

13. Ferrannini E, Natali A: Essential hypertension, metabolic disorders, and insulin resistance. *Am Heart J* 1991;121:1274-1282.

14. Clinical Guidelines on the Identification, Evaluation, and Treatment of Overweight and Obesity in Adults—The Evidence Report. National Institutes of Health. *Obes Res* 1998;6(suppl 2):51S-209S.

15. Thompson PD, Buchner D, Pina IL, et al: Exercise and physical activity in the prevention and treatment of atherosclerotic cardiovascular disease: a statement from the Council on Clinical Cardiology (Subcommittee on Exercise, Rehabilitation, and Prevention) and the Council on Nutrition, Physical Activity, and Metabolism (Subcommittee on Physical Activity). *Circulation* 2003;107:3109-3116.

16. Grundy SM, Hansen B, Smith SC Jr, et al: Clinical management of metabolic syndrome: report of the American Heart Asso-

ciation/National Heart, Lung, and Blood Institute/American Diabetes Association conference on scientific issues related to management. *Circulation* 2004;109:551-556.

17. Appel LJ: Lifestyle modification as a means to prevent and treat high blood pressure. *J Am Soc Nephrol* 2003;14:S99-S102.

18. US Department of Agriculture and US Department of Health and Human Services. Nutrition and your health: dietary guidelines for Americans, 5th ed. Home and Garden Bulletin no. 232. Washington, DC, US Department of Agriculture, 2000, 44 pages.

19. Vega GL, Ma PT, Cater NB, et al: Effects of adding fenofibrate (200 mg/d) to simvastatin (10 mg/d) in patients with combined hyperlipidemia and metabolic syndrome. *Am J Cardiol* 2003;91:956-960.

20. Chobanian AV, Bakris GL, Black HR, et al: The Seventh Report of the Joint National Committee on Prevention, Detection, Evaluation, and Treatment of High Blood Pressure: the JNC 7 report. *JAMA* 2003;289:2560-2572.

21. Reaven G: Insulin resistance, hypertension, and coronary heart disease. *J Clin Hypertens (Greenwich)* 2003;5:269-274.

22. Knowler WC, Barrett-Connor E, Fowler SE, et al: Reduction in the incidence of type 2 diabetes with lifestyle intervention or metformin. *N Engl J Med* 2002;346:393-403.

23. UK Prospective Diabetes Study (UKPDS) Group: Effect of intensive blood-glucose control with metformin on complications in overweight patients with type 2 diabetes. *Lancet* 1998;352:854-865.

24. Dormandy JA, Charbonnel B, Eckland DJ, et al: Secondary prevention of macrovascular events in patients with type 2 diabetes in the PROactive Study (PROspective pioglitAzone Clinical Trial In macroVascular Events): a randomised controlled trial. *Lancet* 2005;366:1279-89.

25. Pearson TA, Blair SN, Daniels SR, et al: AHA Guidelines for Primary Prevention of Cardiovascular Disease and Stroke: 2002 Update: Consensus Panel Guide to Comprehensive Risk Reduction for Adult Patients Without Coronary or Other Atherosclerotic Vascular Diseases. American Heart Association Science Advisory and Coordinating Committee. *Circulation* 2002;106:388-391.

26. Ridker PM, Buring JE, Cook NR, et al: C-reactive protein, the metabolic syndrome, and risk of incident cardiovascular events: an 8-year follow-up of 14,719 initially healthy American women. *Circulation* 2003;107:391-397.

Chapter **2**

Diagnosis
of the Metabolic Syndrome

Although the concept of the metabolic syndrome has existed in various forms for many years, clinical criteria for its diagnosis were not formalized in a way that was useful in clinical practice. Thus, for a long time, the syndrome was recognized by clinical research and pathophysiology, but was not routinely identified in patients.

Recently, attempts have been made to define the criteria that permit a clinical diagnosis of the metabolic syndrome. In 1998 and 1999, a World Health Organization (WHO) committee on diabetes outlined the clinical characteristics required for this diagnosis.[1,2] These criteria were not widely disseminated to the medical community and thus were sparsely applied. More recently, the National Cholesterol Education Program's Adult Treatment Panel III (NCEP ATP III) proposed an updated, different list of criteria (Table 2-1).[3] Because these criteria were linked to widely used clinical guidelines for cholesterol management, they received greater attention. Although ATP III undoubtedly gave the concept a boost, the recommendations were well received because of the increasing prevalence of the metabolic syndrome in the United States. Other criteria for the metabolic syndrome have been proposed and will also be considered in this chapter.

It is important to differentiate between the definition of the metabolic syndrome and the clinical criteria re-

Table 2-1: Diagnosing the Metabolic Syndrome*

Factor	Defining Level
Abdominal obesity	Waist circumference
- Men	≥ 102 cm (≥ 40 in)[†]
- Women	≥ 88 cm (≥ 35 in)
Triglycerides	≥ 150 mg/dL (or on drug treatment for elevated TG)
HDL cholesterol	
- Men	<40 mg/dL
- Women	<50 mg/dL (or on drug treatment for low HDL)
Blood pressure	≥ 130 mm Hg systolic or ≥ 85 mm Hg diastolic (or on drug treatment for high blood pressure)
Fasting glucose	≥ 100 mg/dL (or on drug treatment for elevated glucose)

*From updated NCEP ATP III guidelines.[3]

[†]Lower waist circumference cutpoint (≥90 cm in men and ≥80 cm in women) appears to be appropriate for Asian Americans.

quired for diagnosis. The two are not necessarily the same, and failure to make a distinction has led to confusion. Because the metabolic syndrome is complex, diagnostic criteria must attempt to capture the essence of the condition without necessarily incorporating all of the components. Clinical criteria must also be applicable in daily practice. One limitation of some of the criteria is that they require special testing beyond what is available in routine practice. Special testing may provide additional useful information, but it adds expense and inconvenience that reduce its usefulness in practice. This chapter will focus on clinical criteria for diagnosis, and attempts to develop diagnostic criteria that are useful in routine clinical practice.

ATP III Clinical Criteria

Metabolic Syndrome as a Secondary Target of Therapy in Cholesterol Treatment Guidelines

A primary goal of the NCEP has been to develop evidence-based recommendations for clinical management of high blood cholesterol levels in adults. To date, three Adult Treatment Panel (ATP) reports have been released, the first (ATP I) in 1988.[4] ATP I's justification for advocating cholesterol management was based on epidemiologic evidence, animal studies, limited clinical trial data, and genetic forms of hypercholesterolemia, including genetic disorders of low-density lipoprotein (LDL) metabolism such as familial hypercholesterolemia and polygenic hypercholesterolemia that frequently manifest premature atherosclerotic disease even without other risk factors. Other clinical evidence for cholesterol management included large epidemiologic surveys that had identified a relationship between serum total cholesterol and risk for coronary heart disease (CHD).[5-8] In 1984,[9,10] the Lipid Research Clinic (LRC) Coronary Primary Prevention Trial (CPPT) compared a cholesterol-lowering drug, cholestyramine, to placebo for efficacy in patients with primary hypercholesterolemia. Cholestyramine therapy reduced the primary end point, CHD events, and coronary death. This combined evidence was considered sufficient to warrant inclusion in the NCEP.

Because most of the evidence pointed to LDL cholesterol (LDL-C) as the major atherogenic lipoprotein, ATP I identified LDL-C as the primary target of lipid-lowering therapy. That LDL-C should be the first and major target of therapy was supported in subsequent ATP reports.

In 1993, ATP II retained strong support for LDL lowering through dietary means for primary prevention of CHD. Moreover, a meta-analysis of secondary prevention trials of cholesterol-lowering therapy[11-14] indicated that reducing serum cholesterol was effective in preventing major coronary events and coronary death. The ATP II panel therefore emphasized cholesterol-lowering therapy in patients with established CHD (secondary prevention). Indeed, the panel recommended that LDL-C be reduced to <100 mg/dL in patients with established CHD. ATP II also recommended increased emphasis on obesity and physical inactivity as secondary targets of lipid-lowering therapy. The goal was twofold: (1) to achieve enhanced LDL reduction and (2) to improve other lipid risk factors (ie, low HDL-C and high triglyceride levels). This recommendation was based on growing evidence that low HDL and high triglyceride levels carried atherogenic potential beyond elevated LDL-C.

In 2001, ATP III strengthened the case for LDL-lowering therapy in primary and secondary prevention, based on clinical trials with HMG CoA reductase inhibitors (statins) that showed marked reductions in risk for CHD. Because effective statin therapy was available, recommendations for intensive treatment of LDL-C with drugs were greatly expanded. ATP III emphasized identifying an individual's risk category (Table 2-2). The concept of secondary prevention was extended to high-risk prevention. Patients at high risk have either established CHD or conditions called *CHD risk equivalents*. In other words, if a person without established CHD has a risk for future major coronary events equal to that of someone with CHD, this person is said to have a CHD risk equivalent. Included in this category are patients with clinical forms of atherosclerotic disease (eg, peripheral arterial disease, abdominal aortic aneurysm, and carotid artery disease), patients with diabetes, and those with multiple factors that raise the risk for major coronary events (myo-

Table 2-2: Risk Categories of Adult Treatment Panel III Report

Risk Category	Features of Risk Category
High risk	Established coronary heart disease – peripheral arterial disease – abdominal aortic aneurysm – clinical carotid artery disease – diabetes 2+ major risk factors* and 10-year risk for CHD >20%**
Moderately high risk	2+ major risk factors* and 10-year risk for CHD 10%-20%
Moderate risk	2+ major risk factors* and 10-year risk for CHD <10%**
Lower risk	0-1 risk factor* or 10-year risk for CHD <10%**

* Major risk factors include cigarette smoking, hypertension (blood pressure >140/90 mm Hg or on treatment for hypertension), low HDL cholesterol (<40 mg/dL), family history of premature CHD in first-degree relative (men <55 years; women <60 years), and advancing age (men >45 years; women >55 years).

** 10-year risk for CHD determined by Framingham risk algorithm (see Tables 6-2 and 6-3).

CHD = coronary heart disease

cardial infarction + coronary death) to >20% in 10 years. Evidence indicates that a person with established CHD has a 10-year risk of at least 20% for major coronary events. For high-risk patients (ie, those with CHD or CHD risk equivalents), an LDL-C goal of <100 mg/dL was established. On the basis of recent clinical trials, ATP III guidelines have been updated such that in patients with CHD plus CHD risk equivalents (eg, diabetes) an LDL-C goal of <70 mg/dL is reasonable.[15,16]

ATP III further recognized a risk category called *moderately high risk*, defined as two or more major risk factors plus a 10-year risk for major coronary events of 10% to 20%. The major risk factors other than elevated LDL-C include cigarette smoking; hypertension (blood pressure >140/90 mm Hg or on treatment for hypertension); low HDL cholesterol (HDL-C) (<40 mg/dL); family history of premature CHD in first-degree relative (men <55 years; women <60 years); and advancing age (men >45 years; women >55 years). Diabetes is a major risk factor for CHD, but its presence, in most patients, equates to a CHD risk equivalent.

In ATP III, the 10-year risk for CHD specifies myocardial infarction or coronary death. Estimation of 10-year risk for CHD is made with the Framingham Study risk algorithm. Factors included in this algorithm are cigarette smoking, total cholesterol, HDL-C, blood pressure, and age.

Estimates of 10-year risk can be obtained from Table 2-3 and Table 2-4 or by computer. Computer assessment of risk can be obtained online at www.nhlbi.nih.gov under Cholesterol Guidelines.

For people who have two or more risk factors plus a 10-year risk <10% (moderate risk), the treatment goal for LDL-C is still <130 mg/dL, but drug therapy guidelines are less strict. Most people with 0-1 risk factor (lower risk) have a 10-year risk <10%. Therefore, Framingham risk scoring is not necessary. The LDL-C goal for those with 0-1 risk factor is <160 mg/dL.

Introduction of the Metabolic Syndrome Into ATP III Guidelines

The 1993 ATP II report recognized the high prevalence of obesity and physical inactivity in the United States. It placed increased emphasis on weight reduction in overweight/obese people and increased physical activity in sedentary individuals. Unfortunately, these recommendations had little impact on the cardiovascular community. Therefore, ATP III considered methods to focus attention on obesity and physical inactivity. It identified the metabolic syndrome as a major, complex risk factor that results largely from obesity and sedentary life habits. The ATP III treatment algorithm focused on managing high LDL-C, but once the goals of LDL lowering were attained, attention shifted to the metabolic syndrome and its risk factors. It is important to note that the metabolic syndrome does not include elevated LDL-C, although the two conditions may coexist. For management of the metabolic syndrome, modification of its underlying causes, (ie, overweight/obesity and physical inactivity) took priority.

The introduction of specific criteria for clinical diagnosis of the metabolic syndrome gives the health profession a way to identify patients at increased risk for both atherosclerotic cardiovascular disease (ASCVD) and type 2 diabetes. According to ATP III, patients have the metabolic syndrome if they have three of the five characteristics shown in Table 2-5: qualifying waist circumference (surrogate for abdominal obesity), serum triglyceride levels, HDL cholesterol levels, blood pressure, and plasma glucose. Because each risk factor is a continuous variable, the cut points for each are arbitrary but appear to be typical of patients exhibiting the clustering of metabolic risk factors. Also, because any combination of three of five metabolic risk factors constitutes a diagnosis, risk factor patterns will vary from person to person.

ATP III diagnostic criteria for the metabolic syndrome can be easily identified in clinical practice or in epidemiologic studies, which is a major advantage. ATP III criteria do not capture all features of the syndrome, although growing evidence indicates that most individuals who exhibit the metabolic syndrome according to the ATP III criteria will have most of these features.

Table 2-3: Framingham Point Scores Estimate of 10-Year Risk for Men

Age, years	Points
20-34	-9
35-39	-4
40-44	0
45-49	3
50-54	6
55-59	8
60-64	10
65-69	11
70-74	12
75-79	13

Total cholesterol, mg/dL	Points				
	Age 20-39y	Age 40-49y	Age 50-59y	Age 60-69y	Age 70-79y
<160	0	0	0	0	0
160-199	4	3	2	1	0
200-239	7	5	3	1	0
240-279	9	6	4	2	1
≥280	11	8	5	3	1

	Points				
	Age 20-39y	Age 40-49y	Age 50-59y	Age 60-69y	Age 70-79y
Nonsmoker	0	0	0	0	0
Smoker	8	5	3	1	1

HDL-C, mg/dL	Points
≥60	-1
50-59	0
40-49	1
<40	2

Systolic BP, mm Hg	If untreated	If treated
<120	0	0
120-129	0	1
130-139	1	2
140-159	1	2
≥160	2	3

Point total	10-year risk (%)
<0	<1
0	1
1	1
2	1
3	1
4	1
5	2
6	2
7	3
8	4
9	5
10	6
11	8
12	10
13	12
14	16
15	20
16	25
≥17	≥30

Table 2-4: Framingham Point Scores
Estimate of 10-Year Risk for Women

Age, years	Points
20-34	-7
35-39	-3
40-44	0
45-49	3
50-54	6
55-59	8
60-64	10
65-69	12
70-74	14
75-79	16

Total cholesterol, mg/dL	Points				
	Age 20-39y	Age 40-49y	Age 50-59y	Age 60-69y	Age 70-79y
<160	0	0	0	0	0
160-199	4	3	2	1	1
200-239	8	6	4	2	1
240-279	11	8	5	3	2
≥280	13	10	7	4	2

	Points				
	Age 20-39y	Age 40-49y	Age 50-59y	Age 60-69y	Age 70-79y
Nonsmoker	0	0	0	0	0
Smoker	9	7	4	2	1

HDL-C, mg/dL	Points
≥60	-1
50-59	0
40-49	1
<40	2

Systolic BP, mm Hg	If untreated	If treated
<120	0	0
120-129	1	3
130-139	2	4
140-159	3	5
≥160	4	6

Point total	10-year risk (%)
<9	<1
9	1
10	1
11	1
12	1
13	2
14	2
15	3
16	4
17	5
18	6
19	8
20	11
21	14
22	17
23	22
24	27
≥25	≥30

Table 2-5: ATP III Clinical Identification of the Metabolic Syndrome

A. Risk Factor	B. Defining Level
Abdominal obesity*	Waist circumference**
Men	>102 cm (> 40 in)
Women	>88 cm (> 35 in)
Triglycerides	≥150 mg/dL (or on drug treatment for elevated TG)
HDL cholesterol	
Men	<40 mg/dL
Women	<50 mg/dL (or on drug treatment for low HDL)
Blood pressure	≥130/ ≥85 mm Hg (or on drug treatment for high blood pressure)
Fasting glucose	>100 mg/dL*** (or on drug treatment for elevated glucose)

* Overweight and obesity are associated with insulin resistance and the metabolic syndrome. However, abdominal obesity is more highly correlated with the metabolic risk factors than is an elevated BMI. Therefore, the simple measure of waist circumference is recommended to identify the body weight component of the metabolic syndrome.

** Some male patients can develop multiple metabolic risk factors when their waist circumference is only marginally increased, eg, 94-102 cm (37-39 in). Such patients may have a strong genetic inclination to insulin resistance. Lower waist circumference cut point (≥90 cm in men and ≥80 cm in women) appears to be appropriate for Asian Americans.[3] They should benefit from changes in life habits similarly to men with categoric increases in waist circumference.

*** The American Diabetes Association recently redefined the lower cutpoint for impaired fasting glucose to be >100 mg/dL.[17]

BMI = body mass index

Other components not routinely measured are reported to be common in people with insulin resistance and the metabolic syndrome. These include elevated apolipoprotein B (apo B), small low-density lipoprotein (LDL) particles, insulin resistance and hyperinsulinemia, impaired glucose tolerance, elevated C-reactive protein (CRP), and coagulation factors (eg, PAI-1 and fibrinogen). Although apo B levels often are elevated, LDL-cholesterol levels may not be increased. Their measurement in clinical practice is optional, and we do not now know how their detection will modify clinical management of patients with ATP III criteria for the metabolic syndrome.

World Health Organization Clinical Criteria

In 1998,[1] a WHO consultation group on diabetes classification proposed working criteria for the metabolic syndrome. Table 2-6 summarizes the WHO's 1999 modified proposal, which is available on the WHO Web site.[18] Cardiovascular disease (CVD) is recognized as the primary clinical outcome. A key feature of the WHO metabolic syndrome definition is that insulin resistance is a required constituent.

Acceptable evidence for the metabolic syndrome is one of the following: type 2 diabetes, impaired fasting glucose (IFG), impaired glucose tolerance (IGT), or, for those with normal fasting glucose values (<110 mg/dL), a glucose uptake lower than the lowest quartile for the background population under hyperinsulinemic, euglycemic conditions. Two other risk factors, besides insulin resistance, are sufficient for a diagnosis.

Insulin Resistance

Evidence of insulin resistance is required for the WHO definition because many investigators believe that insulin resistance is at the core of the metabolic syndrome. This idea has been extensively developed by Reaven et al[19-22] and others.[23-25] They hypothesize that insulin resistance might induce other metabolic risk factors. In fact, an alter-

Table 2-6: World Health Organization Clinical Criteria for Metabolic Syndrome*

Insulin resistance, identified by one of the following:

- Type 2 diabetes, impaired fasting glucose
- Impaired glucose tolerance
- For those with normal fasting glucose levels (<110 mg/dL), glucose uptake below the lowest quartile for background population under hyperinsulinemic, euglycemic conditions.

Plus any two of the following:

- Antihypertensive medication and/or high blood pressure (≥140 mm Hg systolic or ≥90 mm Hg diastolic)
- Plasma triglycerides ≥150 mg/dL (≥1.7 mmol/L)
- HDL cholesterol <35 mg/dL (<0.9 mmol/L) in men or <39 mg/dL (1.0 mmol/L) in women
- BMI >30 kg/m^2 and/or waist:hip ratio >0.9 in men, >0.85 in women
- Urinary albumin excretion rate ≥20 μg/min or albumin:creatinine ratio ≥30 mg/g

* World Health Organization: Definition, diagnosis and classification of diabetes mellitus and its complications: Report of a WHO Consultation. Part 1. Diagnosis and classification of diabetes mellitus. Geneva, World Health Organization, 1999 http://whqlibdoc.who.int/hq/1999/WHO_NCD_NCS_99.2.pdf.

HDL = high-density lipoprotein
BMI = body mass index

nate term for the metabolic syndrome is the *insulin resistance syndrome*. According to this hypothesis, obesity is only one cause of insulin resistance. Furthermore, most of the adverse metabolic effects of obesity are thought to be mediated through insulin resistance. This idea differs from that put forth in the ATP III definition, in which insulin resistance is a component of the metabolic syndrome and obesity is the driving force behind the syndrome.

Hyperglycemia often occurs in people with insulin resistance, but it is as much a reflection of decline in insulin secretion as of insulin resistance. Certainly, glucose tolerance testing will improve prediction of type 2 diabetes, but WHO criteria are not likely to enhance prediction of CVD over those of ATP III.

Elevated Blood Pressure

WHO criteria, like those of ATP III, include elevated blood pressure. WHO explicitly lists antihypertensive medication as treatment. ATP III left this indicator out of its list, seemingly inadvertently. The WHO's defining level of blood pressure is higher than that of ATP III. The WHO chose the cut point for categoric hypertension (≥140/90 mm Hg), while ATP III recognized high-normal blood pressure (≥130/85 mm Hg).

Elevated Plasma Triglyceride Levels

The WHO criterion for triglycerides is the same as that of ATP III (ie, levels ≥150 mg/dL). The rationale is also the same.

Reduced HDL Levels

The WHO panel sets lower cut points than does ATP III to define a reduced HDL-C level. For men, the level is <35 mg/dL. ATP III set a higher cut point (<40 mg/dL) because reduction of HDL-C due to obesity in the general male population rarely produces levels as low as 35 mg/dL. When HDL-C levels in men fall below 35 mg/dL, a strong genetic component usually exists. The same is true for women who meet the WHO HDL-C criteria of <39 mg/dL. The ATP III cut point of <50 mg/dL for women represents the 'metabolic' component of lower HDL without the genetic component.

Body Weight

The WHO offered two criteria for body weight indicators: BMI >30 kg/m^2 and waist:hip ratio 0.9 in men and >0.85 in women. In ATP III, BMI was rejected in favor of waist circumference, an indicator of abdominal obesity. Adding the waist:hip ratio is an attempt to include a component of abdominal obesity in the WHO definition. However, most authorities believe that waist circumference is a better indicator of abdominal obesity than is the waist:hip ratio.[26]

Urinary Albumin Level

Urinary microalbuminuria is included in WHO criteria of the metabolic syndrome, for reasons not immediately evident. Microalbuminuria without diabetes presumably indicates 'vascular injury,' which might be considered a consequence of metabolic risk factors. If so, it belongs in an entirely different category of components than the other metabolic risk factors.

European Group for the Study of Insulin Resistance (EGIR)

Authors for the European Group for the Study of Insulin Resistance[27] suggested a modification of WHO criteria for the metabolic syndrome. These criteria are shown in Table 2-7. Insulin resistance was retained as a requirement for the metabolic syndrome and was defined simply as a fasting insulin level in the upper quartile for the population. Other criteria include hyperglycemia, elevated blood pressure, elevated triglyceride levels (and/or reduced HDL-C), and abdominal obesity. The study set a lower cut point for elevated waist circumference (ie, >94 cm in men and >80 cm in women). These criteria have the advantage of simplicity, except for the measurement of fasting insulin. To date, accurate and standardized measurements of fasting insulin are not widely available. Even if

Table 2-7: European Group for the Study of Insulin Resistance

Insulin resistance: upper quartile for fasting insulin level plus two of the following:

- Hyperglycemia (fasting glucose >6.1 mmol/L)
- Blood pressure >140/90 mm Hg
- Serum triglyceride level >2 mmol/L
- HDL cholesterol level <1 mmol/L
- Abdominal obesity: waist circumference for men >94 cm, women >80 cm

they were available, they would be relatively expensive and not routine. Finally, it is not clear that single measurements of fasting insulin levels are a robust surrogate for insulin resistance.

American Association of Clinical Endocrinologists (AACE) Clinical Criteria

The AACE recently offered alternative clinical criteria and a different name for the metabolic syndrome: insulin resistance syndrome.[28] Most investigators equate the metabolic syndrome and the insulin resistance syndrome. However, differences in concept contribute to differences in names. The term *insulin resistance syndrome* signifies the conviction that insulin resistance is the mediating force for all metabolic risk factors. But it further means that insulin resistance is responsible for medical complications beyond the cardiovascular risk factors of the metabolic syndrome. The components of the AACE criteria are shown in Table 2-8. According to the AACE guidelines, a clinical diagnosis of the insulin resistance syndrome

Table 2-8: American Association of Clinical Endocrinologists Clinical Criteria for Diagnosis of the Insulin Resistance Syndrome*

Risk factor components	Cut points for abnormality
Overweight/obesity	BMI >25 kg/m^2
Triglycerides	≥150 mg/dL
Low HDL cholesterol	<40 mg/dL in men <50 mg/dL in women
Elevated blood pressure	≥130/85 mm Hg
2-hour postglucose challenge	>140 mg/dL
Fasting glucose	Between 110 mg/dL and 126 mg/dL
Other risk factors	Family history of type 2 diabetes, hypertension, or CVD Polycystic ovary syndrome Sedentary lifestyle Advancing age Ethnic groups having high risk for type 2 diabetes or CVD

* Diagnosis depends on clinical judgment based on risk factors.
CVD = cardiovascular disease

should be based on clinical judgment, and no specified number of risk factors is required to trigger the diagnosis.

The AACE guidelines propose a lower cut point for body weight than that used in the WHO criteria. A BMI of >25 kg/m^2 includes the categories of both overweight and obesity instead of obesity alone, as in the WHO criteria. The AACE rejected waist circumference, presumably because the recommending committee believed that a lower BMI cut point will be more inclusive of people with excess body weight than waist circumference. In other words, only some overweight people (BMI 25 to 30 kg/m^2) will have abdominal obesity as defined by ATP III. Indeed, it has been estimated that 75% of the adult population in the United States will have a BMI >25 kg/m^2. Hence, most people will have at least one AACE risk factor for the insulin resistance syndrome. The AACE adopted the same criteria as ATP III for elevation of triglyceride levels, reduction of HDL cholesterol levels, and elevation of blood pressure.

The AACE guidelines include IFG (fasting glucose 110-126 mg/dL) and IGT (2-hour postglucose challenge >140 mg/dL). By addition of the latter, the AACE is consistent with WHO criteria, but not with ATP III. ATP III did not include an oral glucose tolerance test (OGTT) because of inconvenience and expense in clinical practice. Furthermore, IGT without IFG was considered by ATP III to provide neither incremental information in predicting CVD risk nor guidance for intervention to reduce this risk. According to NHANES III data,[29] if IGT were to be added to criteria for the diagnosis of the metabolic syndrome, approximately 5% of people older than 50 years would qualify.[30,31] The addition of OGTT by AACE and WHO seemingly is based on two considerations. First, IGT strongly suggests insulin resistance. Second, IGT without IFG denotes a greater risk for diabetes. Both AACE and WHO committees are diabetes-oriented groups. To them, the connection between insulin resistance and development of type 2 diabetes is critically important. The issue of OGTT points out differences in concept of the meaning of the metabolic syndrome (or the insulin resistance syndrome). ATP III focuses mainly on CVD as an outcome of metabolic syndrome, while the WHO and AACE committees shift the priority to predicting type 2 diabetes.

Because the ADA recently reduced the cut point for IFG to 100 mg/dL, fewer people will be found to have IGT without IFG. This could reduce the need for carrying out OGTT.

An important point about the AACE criteria for the insulin resistance syndrome is that once categoric hyperglycemia (type 2 diabetes) intervenes, the diagnosis no longer pertains. One way to view this exclusion is that the insulin resistance syndrome is a risk factor for type 2 diabetes; type 2 diabetes is not a component of the insulin resistance syndrome. This concept differs from that held in both the ATP III and WHO criteria. The latter believe that patients with type 2 diabetes can have the metabolic syndrome if other diagnostic characteristics are present.

Other Features of AACE Insulin Resistance Syndrome

AACE identified these other components of insulin resistance: a family history of type 2 diabetes, hypertension, or CVD; polycystic ovary syndrome; sedentary lifestyle; advancing age; and ethnic groups with high risk for type 2 diabetes. These features are not always accompanied by insulin resistance, but they might be considered risk factors for insulin resistance. Because the AACE diagnosis of the insulin resistance syndrome does not require a specific number of risk factors, these other features can be considered modifiers that can play a role in the clinician's judgment about a given patient.

In 2005, the International Diabetes Federation (IDF)[32] published new clinical criteria for the metabolic syndrome that closely resembled updated ATP III criteria.[3] However, IDF criteria differ from ATP III in that they make the presence of abdominal obesity necessary for diagnosis (Table 2-9). When abdominal obesity is present, two other factors originally listed in the ATP III definition define the metabolic syndrome. For its criteria of abdominal obesity, IDF specified by nationality

Table 2-9: International Diabetes Federation Clinical Criteria for Metabolic Syndrome

Central Obesity (Waist Circumference Ethnicity Specific*)
Plus Any Two of the Following:

- Raised triglycerides: ≥150 mg/dL (1.7 mmol/L) or on specific treatment for this lipid abnormality

- Reduced HDL-cholesterol:
  <40 mg/dL (0.9 mmol/L) in males
  <50 mg/dL (1.1 mmol/L) in females
  or on specific treatment for this lipid abnormality

- Raised blood pressure:
  Systolic ≥130 mm Hg or diastolic ≥85 mm Hg
  or on treatment for previously diagnosed hypertension

- Raised fasting plasma glucose:
  fasting plasma glucose ≥100 mg/dL (5.6 mmol/L)
  or previously diagnosed type 2 diabetes

  If fasting plasma glucose ≥100 mg/dL (5.6 mmol/L), oral glucose tolerance test is strongly recommended to detect type 2 diabetes but not necessarily to define presence of metabolic syndrome.**

* The following waist circumferences were considered lower threshold levels for defining the metabolic syndrome: Europids (peoples of predominantly European origin), Sub-Saharan Africans, Eastern Mediterranean and Middle Eastern (Arab) populations: ≥94 cm (male) and ≥80 cm (female); South Asians, Chinese, Ethnic South and Central Americans: ≥90 cm (male) and ≥80 cm (female); and Japanese ≥85 cm (male) and ≥90 cm (female). If BMI is >30 kg/m^2, central obesity can be assumed and waist circumference does not need to be measured.

** In clinical practice, OGTT to detect IGT is also acceptable, but all reports of the prevalence of the metabolic syndrome should use only the fasting plasma glucose and presence of previously diagnosed diabetes to assess this criterion. Prevalences also incorporating the 2-hour glucose results can be added as supplementary findings.

or ethnicity based on the best available population estimates. For Europeans (or Europid populations), the abdominal obesity was defined as waist circumferences ≥94 cm in men and ≥80 cm in women. For Asian populations, except for Japan, thresholds were ≥90 cm in men and ≥80 cm in women; for Japanese they were ≥80 cm for men and ≥90 cm for women.

Quebec Heart Institute Hypertriglyceridemic Waist

Investigators at the Quebec Heart Institute[33] coined the term *hypertriglyceridemic waist* to indicate a condition with a high risk for ASCVD. This condition has many of the characteristics of the metabolic syndrome. The essential features of hypertriglyceridemic waist are an elevated waist circumference (90 cm or greater) and moderate hypertriglyceridemia (triglyceride concentration 2.0 mmol/L or higher in men). Waist measurements for women have not been specified. Other common features of the condition include a triad of metabolic markers (high insulin and apolipoprotein B levels, and small, dense, LDL particles) and a substantially increased risk of ASCVD.

References

1. Alberti KG, Zimmet PZ: Definition, diagnosis, and classification of diabetes mellitus and its complications, part 1: diagnosis and classification of diabetes mellitus: provisional report of a WHO consultation. *Diabet Med* 1998;15:539-553.

2. Puavilai G, Chanprasertyotin S, Sriphrapradaeng A: Diagnostic criteria for diabetes mellitus and other categories of glucose intolerance: 1997 criteria by the Expert Committee on the Diagnosis and Classification of Diabetes Mellitus (ADA), 1998 WHO consultation criteria, and 1985 WHO criteria. World Health Organization. *Diabetes Res Clin Pract* 1999;44:21-26.

3. Grundy SM, Cleeman JI, Daniels SR, et al: Diagnosis and management of the metabolic syndrome. An American Heart Association/National Heart, Lung and Blood Institute Scientific Statement. *Circulation* 2005;112:2735-2752.

4.   Report of the National Cholesterol Education Program Expert Panel on Detection, Evaluation, and Treatment of High Blood Cholesterol in Adults: the Expert Panel. *Arch Intern Med* 1988;148: 36-69.

5.   Castelli WP, Garrison RJ, Wilson PW, et al: Incidence of coronary heart disease and lipoprotein cholesterol levels. The Framingham Study. *JAMA* 1986;256:2835-2858.

6.   Hulley S, Ashman P, Kuller L, et al: HDL-cholesterol levels in the Multiple Risk Factor Intervention Trial (MRFIT) by the MRFIT Research Group 1,2. *Lipids* 1979;14:119-123.

7.   Stamler J, Wentworth D, Neaton JD: Is relationship between serum cholesterol and risk of premature death from coronary heart disease continuous and graded? Findings in 356,222 primary screenees of the Multiple Risk Factor Intervention Trial (MRFIT). *JAMA* 1986;256:2823-2828.

8.   Horenstein RB, Smith DE, Mosca L: Cholesterol predicts stroke mortality in the Women's Pooling Project. *Stroke* 2002;33:1863-1868.

9.   The Lipid Research Clinics Coronary Primary Prevention Trial results. I. Reduction in incidence of coronary heart disease. *JAMA* 1984;251:351-364.

10.   The Lipid Research Clinics Coronary Primary Prevention Trial results. II. The relationship of reduction in incidence of coronary heart disease to cholesterol lowering. *JAMA* 1984;251:365-374.

11.   Manolio TA, Pearson TA, Wenger NK, et al: Cholesterol and heart disease in older persons and women. Review of an NHLBI workshop. *Ann Epidemiol* 1992;2:161-176.

12.   Silberberg JS, Henry DA: The benefits of reducing cholesterol levels: the need to distinguish primary from secondary prevention. 1. A meta-analysis of cholesterol-lowering trials. *Med J Aust* 1991;155:665-666, 669-670.

13.   Holme I: Cholesterol reduction in single and multifactor randomized trials: relationship to CHD incidence and total mortality as found by meta analysis of twenty-two trials. *Blood Press* 1992; 4:29-34.

14.   Rossouw JE, Lewis B, Rifkind BM: The value of lowering cholesterol after myocardial infarction. *N Engl J Med* 1990;323: 1112-1119.

15.   Grundy SM, Cleeman JI, Merz CN, et al: National Heart, Lung and Blood Institute; American College of Cardiology Foundation;

American Heart Association. Implications of recent clinical trials for the National Cholesterol Education Program Adult Treatment Panel III guidelines. *Circulation* 2004;110:227-239.

16.   Smith SC Jr, Allen J, Blair SN, et al: AHA/ACC guidelines for secondary prevention for patients with coronary and other atherosclerotic vascular disease: 2006 update: endorsed by the National Heart, Lung and Blood Institute. *Circulation* 2006; 113:2363-2372.

17.   The Expert Committee of the Diagnosis and Classification of Diabetes Mellitus: Follow-up report on the diagnosis of diabetes mellitus. *Diabetes Care* 2003;26:3160-3167.

18.   World Health Organization: Definition, diagnosis and classification of diabetes mellitus and its complications: Report of a WHO Consultation. Part 1. Diagnosis and classification of diabetes mellitus. Geneva, World Health Organization, 1999. Available at: http://whqlibdoc.who.int/hq/1999/WHO_NCD_NCS_99.2.pdf. Accessed February 26, 2004.

19.   Reaven GM: Banting lecture 1988. Role of insulin resistance in human disease. *Diabetes* 1988;37:1595-1607.

20.   Reaven GM, Lerner RL, Stern MP, et al: Role of insulin in endogenous hypertriglyceridemia. *J Clin Invest* 1967;46:1756-1767.

21.   Laws A, Reaven GM: Evidence for an independent relationship between insulin resistance and fasting plasma HDL-cholesterol, triglyceride and insulin concentrations. *J Intern Med* 1992; 231:25-30.

22.   Reaven GM, Chen YD, Jeppesen J, et al: Insulin resistance and hyperinsulinemia in individuals with small, dense low density lipoprotein particles. *J Clin Invest* 1993;92:141-146.

23.   Ferrannini E, Haffner SM, Mitchell BD, et al: Hyperinsulinemia: the key feature of a cardiovascular and metabolic syndrome. *Diabetologia* 1991;34:416-422.

24.   Abbasi F, Brown BW Jr, Lamendola C, et al: Relationship between obesity, insulin resistance, and coronary heart disease risk. *J Am Coll Cardiol* 2002;40:937-943.

25.   Bogardus C, Lillioja S, Mott DM, et al: Relationship between degree of obesity and in vivo insulin action in man. *Am J Physiol* 1985;248(3 Pt 1):E286-E291.

26.   National Institutes of Health: Clinical guidelines on the identification, evaluation, and treatment of overweight and obesity trials

in adults—the evidence report. Bethesda, MD, National Heart, Lung, and Blood Institute. NIH Publication no. 98-4083. 1998. 228 pages.

27.   Balkau B, Charles MA: Comment on the provisional report from the WHO consultation. European Group for the Study of Insulin Resistance (EGIR). *Diabet Med* 1999;16:442-433.

28.   Einhorn D, Reaven GM, Cobin RH, et al: American College of Endocrinology position statement on the insulin resistance syndrome. *Endocr Pract* 2003;9:237-252.

29.   Ford ES, Giles WH, Dietz WH: Prevalence of the metabolic syndrome among US adults: findings from the third National Health and Nutrition Examination Survey. *JAMA* 2002;287:356-359.

30.   Meigs JB, Wilson PW, Nathan DM, et al: Prevalence and characteristics of the metabolic syndrome in the San Antonio Heart and Framingham Offspring Studies. *Diabetes* 2003;52:2160-2167.

31.   Grundy SM, Brewer HB Jr, Cleeman JI, et al: Definition of metabolic syndrome: Report of the National Heart, Lung, and Blood Institute/American Heart Association conference on scientific issues related to definition. *Circulation* 2004;109:433-438.

32.   Alberti KG, Zimmet P, Shaw J: IDF Epidemiology Task Force Consensus Group. The metabolic syndrome—a new worldwide definition. *Lancet* 2005;366:1059-2062.

33.   Lemieux I, Pascot A, Couillard C, et al: Hypertriglyceridemic waist: A marker of the atherogenic metabolic triad (hyperinsulinemia; hyperapolipoprotein B; small, dense LDL) in men? *Circulation* 2000;102:179-184.

Chapter **3**

Treatment and Prevention Through Lifestyle Modification

The promotion of lifestyle changes should be the first-line approach to management or prevention of the metabolic syndrome. Specific guidelines have been developed for treatment of major risk factors, and these may require drug therapies. However, adoption of lifestyle changes, particularly before atherosclerotic cardiovascular disease (ASCVD) and diabetes have developed, can go a long way toward the prevention of these complications.

Although unalterable genetic factors affect each person, the right combination and intensity of lifestyle improvements can have a significant impact on outcome. For this reason, and the fact that an estimated one fourth of all Americans are at risk for or already have significant manifestations of the metabolic syndrome, a public health approach promises the greatest good for the greatest number.

Behavioral Changes

An effective nonpharmacologic, behavioral approach to reducing the impact of the metabolic syndrome on health combines four targets: smoking cessation, weight loss, increased physical activity, and dietary modification. The ultimate goal is an entirely new lifestyle, something that is unlikely to be achieved by anything other than a progressive approach, one step at a time. Fortu-

Table 3-1: Behavioral Changes for a Better Lifestyle

Goal	Requirements	Time to completion
Weight loss	10% reduction in body weight in 1 year	1.5 lb/wk
Quit smoking	Freedom	30 days
Diet optimization	ATP III guidelines	60 days
Exercise	Regular routine at least 30 min 5 x/wk at 80% maximum pulse rate	Check calendar diary for compliance every month
Clear kitchen of junk food	None left	Tomorrow

nately, each step carries its own rewards, so that the motivation that is all-important in pursuing the goal can be reinforced at each interval.

A behavioral modification program is based on the urgency of modifying each behavior, the patient's motivation to do so, the support and follow-through available, and the patient's overall health status. Patients should be encouraged to design an overall program at the outset, complete with a reasonable timetable for each phase—a master plan, if you will. Setting a goal, having it in writing, and maintaining a commitment offer real benefits (Table 3-1).

How to Achieve Behavioral Changes

Physicians should emphasize the lifestyle changes set forth by Adult Treatment Panel III (ATP III) as the first and most important intervention for patients with or at risk for the metabolic syndrome.

The physician's participation is required for behavior modification success. The patient will look to the physician for guidance, but equally important, the physician's attitude is crucial. Unfortunately, many physicians have a negative attitude about the prospects for behavior modification. They tend to be overly influenced by those patients who fail to make meaningful changes. But millions of people have successfully modified their life habits to improve their health, including patients who have stopped smoking, have started and maintained an exercise program, or have successfully lost weight. For these reasons, a positive and encouraging outlook is essential. Physician participation in behavior modification requires a few minutes with the patient to take a proper history and make the appropriate referrals. For healthy adults, a serum lipoprotein panel should be obtained at least once every 5 years. Blood pressure levels should be measured every 2 years, or more frequently for elevations, as outlined in JNC 7. If a person has two or more major risk factors, Framingham Heart Study risk scoring should be performed.

Weight Reduction

Goal of Therapy

A defined goal of weight reduction should be set for overweight/obese patients with the metabolic syndrome.[1,2] Clinical trials indicate that a reasonable goal is to achieve a reduction in body weight of 10% in 6 months to 1 year. For example, a person who weighs 220 lb should strive to reduce his or her weight to 200 lb in the first year. Then, a decision can be made on whether further weight loss is required. The decision will be based primarily on the response in metabolic risk factors. Studies have shown that much of the benefit of reducing these risk factors can be achieved with the reduction of 10% of body weight, which is realistic and practical for many patients.

Low-Calorie Diets

A reduction in caloric intake is required for weight reduction. There have been two persistent questions about such diets: (1) how low should the calorie count be? and (2) what should be the composition of a low-calorie diet in obese people?

To achieve a weight loss of about 25 lb in 6 months, it is necessary to reduce caloric intake by about 500 calories per day. This change will result in a weight reduction of approximately 1 pound per week.[1,2] Many people, however, desire to 'jump-start' the weight reduction process. They prefer to reduce calories by about 1,000 calories per day. To get this jump-start, women should reduce calories to a maximum of 1,200 per day, and men should not exceed 1,800 calories per day. The downside of extreme reduction in calories is that the focus is placed more on caloric deficit than on behavior modification. Only through behavior modification will it be possible to achieve long-term weight reduction. Therefore, more emphasis should be placed on behavior modification than on calorie counting for long-term weight reduction.

Many 'weight reduction' diets are advocated and promoted. Most of these are extreme diets that emphasize rapid weight reduction. They are not the types of diet that people can follow for the rest of their lives. Some of these diets are very low in fat. Others promote reduction of carbohydrates. A diet that is reduced in fat and carbohydrates so that the relative amounts left in the diet are balanced is preferred. Thus, even if a major caloric deficit is used to jump-start the process, a combined reduction of fats and carbohydrates will make it easier to achieve a long-term, healthy diet.

Increased Physical Activity as a Weight Reduction Adjunct

Including increased exercise in a weight-reduction regimen offers several advantages.[1,2] As examined later in the chapter, exercise helps to mitigate the metabolic risk factors in addition to its effect on weight reduction. Furthermore, it promotes energy expenditure and can contribute 2% to 3% of body weight reduction.

Weight Reduction Drugs

Two types of weight reduction drugs are available for clinical use.[1] One is an appetite suppressant; the other reduces fat absorption. The only approved drug to inhibit appetite is sibutramine (Meridia®), a serotonin and noradrenaline reuptake inhibitor. Sibutramine generally is well tolerated, though in some patients it causes dry mouth, anorexia, and insomnia. The major concern is in patients with hypertension; it can raise blood pressure, which is worrisome in patients at risk for ASCVD. In short-term trials of weight-reduction diets, sibutramine can produce an additional 5% reduction in body weight in more than half the subjects. An unresolved question is whether it can be used for a lifetime. Clinical trials have been too short to answer this question. Therefore, long-term trials are required to determine its place in the treatment of obesity.

Orlistat (Xenical®) inhibits the absorption of fat, operating in the gut to inhibit intestinal lipase. Unhydrolyzed dietary fat cannot be absorbed and consequently is excreted. When given at the recommended dose (120 mg 3 times daily), this drug reduces fat absorption by approximately 30%. Short-term clinical trials show that orlistat will reduce body weight about 4% beyond what can be achieved by low-calorie diets. Fat malabsorption (steatorrhea) is an unacceptable side effect in some patients. Again, whether efficacy and tolerability persist over many years has not been tested.

Bariatric Surgery

Gastrointestinal (GI) surgery to produce weight loss has gained popularity among some obese patients in the United States. Many patients choose bariatric surgery because they may feel socially rejected and psychologically depressed, or as part of a regimen to help cope with severe medical problems, such as diabetes. Rapid weight reduction in obese people greatly increases the risk for gallstone formation. Careful, thorough evaluation of patients for bariatric surgery is required. Selection of patients for surgery should follow existing guidelines.[3]

Diet Composition
During and After Weight Reduction

Millions of overweight people commonly believe that if they could just find the 'right' diet they would lose weight. This view is bolstered and promoted by commercial interests. Through the years, many diet books have been advertised and sold. Most of the recommended diets are extreme, restrictive, and favor the use of just a few foods or types of foods. Two currently popular are low-fat diets and low-carbohydrate diets. Others identify a small range of 'acceptable' foods. Unfortunately, most people who adopt extreme diets regain the weight they lose. The claim that extreme diets are useful to jump-start successful weight reduction has not been proved.

As a rule, the composition of a weight reduction diet should resemble as closely as possible the diet that the patient will eventually follow daily. Behavior modification should begin immediately, and the patient's acquired eating habits should be used in the long run as well as the short run.

In choosing a short-term and long-term eating pattern, a few principles should be followed.[1,4] Because obesity typically is accompanied by eating too much fat and carbohydrates, both need to be reduced, especially animal fats, because they raise the serum cholesterol level. Vegetable oils or soft margarines are preferable. There are many sources of excessive carbohydrates in the diet of obese people. These should be identified and reduced or avoided. The diet should be liberal in fruits and vegetables. The fat percentage in the diet depends on personal preference; it can range from 25% to 35% of calories.

Whether patients are following a weight-reduction diet or a weight-maintenance diet, a few principles should be observed for diet composition. These are summarized, with the rationale for the recommendations.

Saturated fats. In cross-population studies, higher intakes of saturated fats are accompanied by increased risk for ASCVD. The reason appears to be that saturated fats raise the serum low-density lipoprotein (LDL)-cholesterol level, one of the chief culprits for cardiovascular disease.[5] A 1% change in saturated fatty acid intake in either direction will produce a corresponding 1% to 2% change in serum cholesterol level, making saturated fats a major determinant of LDL cholesterol levels.[5,6] Although it is not possible to remove all saturated fats from the diet, intake should be reduced to less than 10% of total calories for the general public and to less than 7% for people at risk for ASCVD. The major sources of saturated fats in the diet are dairy products (butter, whole milk, cheese, ice cream, cream); animal fats (lard, tallow, marbled meat, hamburger, ground meat); processed meats (sausage, salami, frankfurters, bologna); tropical oils (palm oil, coconut oil, and palm kernel oil); baked products and mixed dishes containing dairy fat and tropical oils.

Trans fats. These fats are unsaturated but have a double bond in the trans configuration. They are produced by hydrogenation of polyunsaturated oils, a process that raises their melting points and turns liquids into solids at room temperature. The trans fats raise LDL-cholesterol levels similarly to saturated fatty acids.[5,6] The typical American diet contains 2% to 4% of total calories as trans fatty acids. Common sources of trans fatty acids are shortenings and hard margarines; bakery goods made with shortenings (cakes and pies); foods prepared with shortenings (eg, French fries); and milk fat.

Dietary cholesterol. The third LDL-raising nutrient of the diet is cholesterol. The American diet normally contains 300 to 500 mg/d of cholesterol. A cholesterol-lowering diet for the general public should be reduced to <300 mg/d, but people at risk for ASCVD should reduce intake to <200 mg/d. The major sources of dietary cholesterol are egg yolks (240 mg/egg); dietary fats (especially milk fat products); and meat. In a typical American diet, intake of dietary cholesterol is about equally divided among these three sources.

Unsaturated fats. The harmless unsaturated fats are of three types: *cis*-monounsaturated, N-6 polyunsaturated, and N-3 polyunsaturated. The typical American diet contains 25% to 30% of total calories as unsaturated fats. Unsaturated fats do not raise the LDL-cholesterol level and thus are preferred over saturated fats. Animal fats are rich in monounsaturated fats, so when saturated animal fats are reduced, monounsaturated fats are, too. In the Mediterranean region, which has a high intake of monounsaturated fat (olive oil), the prevalence of ASCVD is low.[7]

The other major source of unsaturated fats is plant oils. Oils that are particularly rich in monounsaturated fatty acids include olive oil, canola oil, and high-oleic safflower oil.

N-6 polyunsaturated fats are derived exclusively from plant sources. Clinical trials have shown that enriching the diet with N-6 polyunsaturated fats at the expense of saturated fats will produce lower serum cholesterol levels and fewer major coronary events.[8] Usual sources are corn oil, safflower oil, and soybean oil.

N-3 polyunsaturated fatty acids can come from either fish oils or plant oils. The N-3 polyunsaturates in fish oil consist of eicosapentaenoic acid (EPA) (20:5) and docosahexaenoic acid (DHA) (22:6). Those from plant oils consist mostly of linolenic acid. The diet normally contains about 1% of total calories as N-3 fatty acids. These fatty acids may have special biologic properties that may protect against ASCVD or its complications and are now under study.[8]

Carbohydrates. There are two main types of carbohydrates: sugars (monosaccharides and disaccharides) and polysaccharides (starches and fiber). The typical diet contains 45% to 55% of calories as carbohydrates. Although it was previously thought that high intake of carbohydrates is without adverse effects, recent evidence suggests that overconsumption of carbohydrates contributes to obesity.[8] Moreover, high-carbohydrate diets can raise triglyceride levels, reduce high-density lipoprotein (HDL) cholesterol levels, and enhance postprandial responses to glucose and insulin.[7]

To prevent these responses and to promote weight control, patients must pay attention to the sources of carbohydrates. Some investigators have identified particular carbohydrate-rich foods that may give an exaggerated postprandial glucose response. These foods are called high-glycemic index foods. These include bread, processed cereals, cookies and crackers, potatoes, and rice. Even so, when these foods are consumed in mixed-food meals, some of their hyperglycemic action may be attenuated.

Common sources of excess sugar in the diet are soft drinks, fruit juices, cookies, cakes, pies, honey, and syrup. Simple sugars are also present in skim milk and fruits, although potentially useful nutrients are contained in these foods as well. Common sources of excess polysaccharides are rice, bread, potatoes, pasta, and grains. Many nutritionists prefer whole grains as a carbohydrate source because they contain fiber as well as digestible starch. High intake of fiber is widely advocated because it can reduce the glycemic response and may lower serum cholesterol levels.

Good sources of high-fiber foods are fruits, vegetables, whole grains, dried beans, and oat bran. Psyllium bulk laxatives are also a good source of fiber.

Protein. Many animal and plant products are good sources of protein, such as lean meats and skim milk. Sources of animal protein that are lower in saturated fat and cholesterol include fat-free and low-fat dairy products, egg whites, fish, skinless poultry, and lean meats. Soy and other vegetable proteins can supply adequate nutrition without the accompanying animal fats. Despite claims to the contrary, the amount and quality of protein have little effect on plasma LDL-C levels.

Plant stanols/sterols. Esters of plant stanols and sterols at dosages of 2 g/d can lower LDL-C levels by 6% to 15% when incorporated into margarines and similar fat-containing products.[9] Stanol esters are preferable to sterol esters because they are absorbed to a lesser extent. Plant stanol esters can be recommended as part of an LDL-lowering diet.

Antioxidants. Studies of the antioxidants ascorbic acid (vitamin C), α-tocopherol (vitamin E), β-carotene, ubiquinone (coenzyme Q10), bioflavonoids, and selenium in cardiovascular disease have produced mixed results, even though oxidation of LDL appears to be an important step in the development of atherosclerosis. Population studies support the contention that diets rich in fruits, vegetables, and other foods high in antioxidants are associated with decreased risk of CHD. Controlled clinical trials, however, have been equivocal. On the basis of results in laboratory animals and small clinical studies, antioxidants appear to offer potential for long-term reduction of risk for ASCVD.

Alcohol. Observational, case-control, cohort, and ecologic studies indicate a J-curve relationship between alcohol consumption and CHD risk. These studies indicate that 1/2 to 1 oz of ethanol a day in any form is associated with lower risk for CHD.[10,11] Whether alcohol prevents CHD remains uncertain. Because higher doses are convincingly associated with substantial risk of multiple disease states, health claims for alcohol, if any, must be disseminated with great care to a nation of 20 million to 30 million people suffering from alcohol abuse.

Sodium, potassium, and calcium. Lowering salt intake to 2,400 mg or 1,800 mg/d can lower blood pressure and may reduce risk for hypertension.[12-14] The diet that contains many of the benefits listed above—high in fruits and vegetables, low-fat dairy products, whole grains, poultry, fish, and nuts and low in fats, red meat, and sweets—is also rich in potassium, calcium, and magnesium. Such a diet lowers blood pressure even without a change in salt intake.[14]

Neutraceuticals. There is great public interest in the neutraceuticals, as well as in complementary and alternative medicine. Unfortunately, accumulating convincing evidence in a field as complex as the metabolic syndrome requires enormous expenditures of time, effort, and money. Disinterested parties, such as the National Institutes of Health, are just beginning to explore gathering the necessary data to investigate the claimed benefits of neutraceuticals.

Physical Activity

Physical inactivity is a major risk factor for CHD.[15] Every component of the metabolic syndrome benefits from exercise. Lipid levels improve; HDL is elevated; VLDL is lowered, and often, LDL is also lowered. Blood pressure falls; insulin resistance declines; glycogen synthesis and insulin-stimulated glucose uptake are enhanced;[16] insulin-independent glucose transport increases; and cardiovascular capacity increases along with coronary blood flow. At the same time, morphologic changes and increased capillary supply in muscle tissue shift fuel requirements to fat, reducing glycolytic flux and acid-base fluctuations. Taken collectively, these adaptations result in enhanced performance capacity and lower demands on insulin/glucose metabolism.[17]

Most people can devise their own exercise programs with minimal guidelines from health professionals. Perhaps the most important advice concerns duration and intensity. The minimum effort to improve cardiovascular fitness appears to be in the range of 30 minutes of exercise 4 to 5 times a week at 70% of age-adjusted maximum pulse rate. Clinicians can advise 30 minutes of brisk walking or raking leaves, 15 minutes of running,

Table 3-2: Caloric Expenditure by Activity

Activity	Cal/h	Activity	Cal/h
Sleep	80	Biking	210
Sitting	100	Walking	210
Driving	120	Gardening	220
Fishing	130	Golf	250
Standing	140	Swimming	300
Housework	180	Jogging	585

or 45 minutes of playing volleyball on most, if not all, days of the week. Maximum heart rate can be calculated by this formula:

Women	**Men**
209 minus age x 0.7	214 minus age x 0.8

Wrist pulse monitors are available commercially. A few patients, such as those with autonomic neuropathy from diabetes, cannot increase their pulse rates normally and require expert exercise counseling to establish a safe and effective routine. Patients with cardiac disease or other limitations on physical activity will benefit from professional exercise advice to devise the safest and most effective programs.

One rule about exercise applies universally: 'If you don't like it, you won't do it.' Tips to increase activity include parking farther away from your destination and walking, using stairs instead of elevators, using hand-operated tools instead of power tools (eg, lawnmowers), and finding an active hobby such as swimming or tennis. The caloric expenditure for a variety of activities is listed in Table 3-2.

Table 3-3: Tobacco-related Health Problems

- A smoker is 2 to 6 times more likely to have a heart attack or stroke; the greater the tobacco use, the higher the risk.

- Smoking increases risk for cancers of the mouth, larynx, pharynx, esophagus, lung, stomach, pancreas, kidney, breast, bladder, and cervix.

- Respiratory diseases linked to tobacco use include chronic obstructive pulmonary disease, emphysema, chronic bronchitis, bronchial asthma, and hay fever.

- Surgeons found poorer healing among smokers; some will not perform spinal fusion on smokers because their spines do not fuse. Some plastic surgeons refuse to perform cosmetic surgery on smokers because of poor results.

- Female smokers have a unique set of risks:
  - Smoking greatly elevates the risk of heart attack and stroke in women taking birth-control pills.

  - Women who smoke during pregnancy are more likely to have a miscarriage, stillbirth, or baby with a low birth weight.

  - There is a direct relationship between smoking during pregnancy and sudden infant death syndrome (SIDS).

  - Smoking in pregnancy may be responsible for as many as 10% of all infant deaths in the United States.

- Female smokers, etc. *(continued)*
  - Other increased risks for female smokers include high blood pressure and circulation problems, and an increased risk of developing osteoporosis and its attendant risk for bone fractures.
- Men experience more erectile dysfunction and impotence.
- Additional associated conditions for *both* sexes include:
  - Gastroesophageal reflux disease, peptic ulcer disease, and ulcerative colitis
  - Renal diseases
  - Age-related macular degeneration, glaucoma, and cataract
  - Gingivitis and periodontal diseases
  - Gray hair and baldness
  - Premature wrinkles
  - Infertility in men and women
  - Weakened immune system
  - Sore eyes, sore throat
  - Headaches
  - Overall decreased life expectancy

Table 3-4: Methods That Sometimes Help Patients to Stop Smoking

- Nicotine replacement—pills, patches, and lozenges in a variety of formulations and dosing schedules aim to replace the addictive chemical in tobacco, breaking the multiple social and habit patterns associated with smoking before weaning the smoker from the drug itself. Nicotine replacement is an effective addition to smoking cessation programs and has been credited with a significant success rate.

- Tapering—as with any addiction, stringing out withdrawal allows the body to readapt to its drug-free state gradually, with fewer symptoms. A rigid schedule is required, and intense personal monitoring greatly enhances the success rate. One recommended schedule is to ration a declining daily number of cigarettes each morning and lock up the rest.

Smoking Cessation

There is little disagreement on the overriding importance of smoking cessation in preventing cardiovascular disease. Tobacco is the leading preventable cause of death and disease in the United States. The literature is full of examples of the benefits of smoking cessation. Cigarette smoke contains more than 4,000 chemicals, including ammonia, arsenic, carbon monoxide, DDT, formaldehyde, and nitric acid. At least three of these compounds are known carcinogens. To date, tobacco has been identified as the cause of, or a major contributor to, 29 diseases, including ASCVD. Table 3-3 is a comprehensive list of tobacco-related health problems.[18]

- Bupropion (Zyban®) has been approved by the Food and Drug Administration for smoking cessation. How Zyban® works is largely unknown, but it claims a 1-year success rate of 30% in a comprehensive cessation program, and 35% when nicotine replacement is added.[18]
- Pearls:
  - Cost—a patient's motivation can be increased by calculating the cost of the patient's smoking habit.
  - Halfway measure—one of the best ideas to initiate a cessation program is to encourage the smoker to throw away half of each cigarette. Many of the toxins in tobacco are removed by the filter as the smoke passes through it, so the second half of the cigarette is far more pathogenic than the first half. Ask the patient to draw a line around the middle of each cigarette and discard it after smoking to the line.

Nicotine is addictive. Withdrawal symptoms may last for weeks. Addicts who have successfully abandoned cocaine, heroin, amphetamines, psychedelics, and sedatives still have difficulty giving up smoking. On the brighter side, many smokers have been able to quit, using one or more of the many available methods.

The principal ingredient behind all successful smoking programs is motivation. Repetition is the keystone to effective motivation. There is no better place to start than showing a patient the list of smoking-related diseases (Table 3-3). Fear motivates—perhaps it is the most effective motivator. A list of methods that have been shown to be effective in smoking cessation appears in Table 3-4.

To convince patients that smoking cessation is necessary, the clinician must overcome their objections. Perhaps the greatest obstacle, particularly in overweight patients, is the patient's fear of weight gain. Eighty percent of quitters will gain an average of 4.5 to 7 lb, but 13% of women and 10% of men will gain more than 28 lb.[19,20] Women are particularly intimidated by this problem. The best and perhaps only response to this objection is simply that smoking is a greater risk to health in many more ways than excess body weight. A third of the weight gain associated with smoking cessation appears to be caused by a decrease in the resting metabolic rate of 100 cal/d.[21] The remaining two thirds comes from increased caloric intake, the result of improved ability to taste food. This weight gain is more resistant to dietary counseling than other forms of overweight. Various drugs, including nicotine phenylpropanolamine and bupropion, delay postcessation weight gain, but their effect does not persist after discontinuation.

Long-term weight loss is possible. A key decision to make is whether to institute weight loss and smoking cessation simultaneously or sequentially.

Public Health Approach

The goals of the public health approach to preventing ASCVD and diabetes are fourfold: foster healthy eating habits, encourage weight control, tout the benefits of physical activity, and strongly advocate for the avoidance of smoking and for smoking cessation. Much of the reduction in ASCVD in the United States in the past 50 years can be ascribed to the success of the public health approach. Smoking among men has declined by almost half. The intake of animal fats and cholesterol, chief components of an unhealthy diet, have declined substantially. Both changes have contributed to reducing ASCVD. Unfortunately, the rise in obesity and sedentary habits of Americans have had the opposite effect on the prevalence of the metabolic syndrome and type 2 diabetes. While the dietary and smoking messages need constant reinforcement, the problems of obesity and lack of exercise constitute a public health crisis. Consequently, all of the approaches to public health education need to be mobilized: government, media, academia, educational institutions, industry, and health organizations.

References

1. National Institutes of Health: Clinical guidelines on the identification, evaluation, and treatment of overweight and obesity in adults—the evidence report. Bethesda, MD, National Heart, Lung, and Blood Institute. NIH Publication no. 98-4083. 1998. 228 pages.

2. Grundy SM, Hansen B, Smith SC Jr, et al: Clinical management of metabolic syndrome: report of the American Heart Association/National Heart, Lung, and Blood Institute/American Diabetes Association conference on scientific issues related to management. *Circulation* 2004;109:551-556.

3. NIH conference. Gastrointestinal surgery for severe obesity. Consensus Development Conference Panel. *Ann Intern Med* 1991; 115:956-961.

4. The periodic health examination: age-specific charts. US Preventive Services Task Force. *Am Fam Physician* 1990;41:189-204.

5. Grundy SM, Denke MA: Dietary influences on serum lipids and lipoproteins. *J Lipid Res* 1990;31:1149-1172.

6. Mensink RP, Katan MB: Effects of dietary fatty acids on serum lipids and lipoproteins: A meta-analysis of 27 trials. *Arterioscler Thromb* 1992;12:911-919.

7. Grundy SM: The optimal ratio of fat-to-carbohydrate in the diet. *Annu Rev Nutr* 1999;19:325-341.

8. US Department of Agriculture, US Department of Health and Human Services: Nutrition and your health: dietary guidelines for Americans. 5th ed. Washington, DC, US Department of Agriculture. Home and Garden Bulletin no. 232. 2000. 44 pages.

9. Hallikainen MA, Uusitupa MI: Effects of 2 low-fat stanol ester-containing margarines on serum cholesterol concentrations as part of a low-fat diet in hypercholesterolemic subjects. *Am J Clin Nutr* 1999;69:403-410.

10.   Criqui MH: Alcohol and coronary heart disease: consistent relationship and public health implications. *Clinica Chimica Acta* 1996;246:51-57.

11.   Dufour MC: If you drink alcoholic beverages do so in moderation: what does this mean? *J Nutr* 2001;131(2S-1):552S-561S.

12.   The sixth report of the Joint National Committee on prevention, detection, evaluation, and treatment of high blood pressure. *Arch Intern Med* 1997;157:2413-2446.

13.   Chobanian AV, Bakris GL, Black HR, et al: Seventh report of the Joint National Committee on Prevention, Detection, Evaluation, and Treatment of High Blood Pressure. *Hypertension* 2003;42:1206-1252.

14.   Appel LJ, Moore TJ, Obarzanek E, et al: A clinical trial of the effects of dietary patterns on blood pressure. DASH Collaborative Research Group. *N Engl J Med* 1997;336:1117-1124.

15.   Fletcher GF, Balady G, Blair SN, et al: Statements on exercise: benefits and recommendations for physical activity programs for all Americans: a statement for health professionals by the Committee on Exercise and Cardiac Rehabilitation of the Council on Clinical Cardiology, American Heart Association. *Circulation* 1996;94:857-862.

16.   Sakamoto K, Goodyear LJ: Invited review: intracellular signaling in contracting skeletal muscle. *J Appl Physiol* 2002;93:369-383.

17.   US Department of Health and Human Services: Physical activity and health: a Report of the Surgeon General. Atlanta, Georgia: US Department of Health and Human Services, Centers for Disease Control and Prevention, National Center for Chronic Disease Prevention and Health Promotion, 1996, 278 pages.

18.   Klesges RC, Meyers AW, Klesges LM, et al: Smoking, body weight, and their effects on smoking behavior: a comprehensive review of the literature. *Psychol Bull* 1989;106:204-230.

19.   Williamson DI, Madans J, Anda RI, et al: Smoking cessation and severity of weight gain in a national cohort. *N Engl J Med* 1991;34:739-745.

20.   Pomerleau GS, Kurth CL: Willingness of female smokers to tolerate postcessation weight gain. *J Subst Abuse* 1996;8:371-378.

21.   Gilbert RM, Pope MA: Early effects of quitting smoking. *Psychopharmacology (Berl)* 1982;78:121-127.

Chapter **4**

Type 2 Diabetes, Hypertension, and Atherogenic Dyslipidemia: Pharmacologic Treatment Options

Most people with type 2 diabetes have the metabolic syndrome, a heterogeneous condition consisting of several risk factors of varying severity. One risk factor is elevated plasma glucose, which, in its more severe forms, is called diabetes. Impairment of insulin secretion by pancreatic β cells also usually coexists with insulin resistance in clinically elevated glucose. In the presence of insulin resistance, the degree of glucose elevation depends largely on the severity of the defect in insulin secretion. This chapter examines the clinical approach to three levels of glucose elevation associated with the metabolic syndrome: impaired glucose tolerance (IGT), impaired fasting glucose (IFG), and categoric hyperglycemia (diabetes). IGT and IFG will be used synonymously with prediabetes.

Definitions

Guidelines for the classification and diagnosis of diabetes continue to evolve. Type 2 diabetes is a complex condition of which hyperglycemia is only one component. However, diabetes is conventionally equated with hyperglycemia.

If hyperglycemia is to be used as the defining parameter of type 2 diabetes, a clinical cutoff point must be determined. Two measures have been proposed: fasting hyperglycemia and postprandial hyperglycemia. The latter is typically determined by oral glucose tolerance testing (OGTT). The American Diabetes Association (ADA) does not recommend OGTT to diagnose diabetes and has instead adopted fasting hyperglycemia as the critical measure.

The defining level for a diabetes diagnosis relates to the glucose level that will produce microvascular disease if maintained for a long period. Previously, a fasting plasma glucose level of >140 mg/dL was the defining characteristic. Recently, the ADA lowered the threshold to >126 mg/dL.[1]

The World Health Organization (WHO) task force on diabetes classification favors the use of postprandial glucose levels for the diagnosis of diabetes.[2] The WHO cut-off point is a 2-hour glucose level >200 mg/dL. This approach may more reliably identify people at risk for microvascular disease. However, some patients with an abnormal OGTT will be normoglycemic or have only IFG on fasting samples. The benefit of OGTT is that it allows earlier identification of diabetes and can lead to more aggressive risk reduction early in the course of the disease. The major drawbacks are the test's cost and inconvenience.

Goals of Therapy

The ultimate goal of therapy for type 2 diabetes is to prevent its complications, particularly macrovascular and microvascular disease. Macrovascular disease takes the various forms of classic atherosclerotic cardiovascular disease (ASCVD), and prevention is achieved mainly by control of the risk factors for cardiovascular disease (CVD), such as hyperglycemia, dyslipidemia, hypertension, and a prothrombotic state. Microvascular complications include diabetic eye disease, chronic renal failure, and nephropathy. Control of elevated plasma glucose is paramount in preventing microvascular disease. The ADA publishes guidelines for glucose control,[3] and patients with type 2 diabetes should self-monitor their glucose levels.

Fasting, preprandial, and bedtime glucose levels should be kept below 140 mg/dL. Ideally, fasting levels should be below 115 mg/dL. Hemoglobin A_{1c} levels should be maintained below 7%.

The Metabolic Syndrome as a Risk Factor for Type 2 Diabetes

There are two concomitant causes of type 2 diabetes: insulin resistance and defective insulin secretion. Insulin resistance usually precedes the onset of defective insulin secretion by many years. Most people with the metabolic syndrome are insulin resistant, which makes their risk for ultimately developing type 2 diabetes approximately five-fold higher than that of people without the metabolic syndrome.[4] This higher risk exists even when the fasting glucose level is not elevated and glucose tolerance is normal.

First-line therapy for the metabolic syndrome is life-style changes, primarily weight reduction and increased physical activity. The goal of lifestyle therapy is twofold: to reduce the risk for ASCVD and to reduce the risk for type 2 diabetes. Drug therapies that target the metabolic risk factors may be required to prevent ASCVD. However, drug therapy is not indicated for prevention of type 2 diabetes when fasting and postprandial glucose levels are in the normal range.

Therapeutic Reduction in Risk for Type 2 Diabetes

Drug therapies

The United States Diabetes Prevention Program[5] has demonstrated that metformin (Glucophage®) therapy will significantly reduce the risk for new-onset diabetes in patients with IGT/IFG. However, its findings raise several major questions. First, does delaying the onset of type 2 diabetes in patients with IGT/IFG modify their long-term prognosis? Second, is diabetes prevention cost-effective? The cost of this therapy per year of life saved has not been adequately evaluated. Third, can our health-care system afford the added burden of paying for diabetes prevention with drug therapy, even if it is medically worthwhile? Fourth, is drug therapy safe enough to justify its use? Metformin appears to be relatively safe. However, the long-term safety of thiazolidinediones (TZDs), which may be considered preventive therapy, has not been fully documented. Also, the costs of TZDs are a factor. Because these questions have not been adequately answered, current treatment recommendations do not support the use of drug therapies to prevent type 2 diabetes in people with IGT/IFG.

Treatment of Diabetes

Treatment of Cardiovascular Risk Factors

Treating the risk factors associated with macrovascular disease, such as atherogenic dyslipidemia and hypertension, will reduce ASCVD risk in diabetic patients as well as in nondiabetic ones. Treatment with HMG-CoA reductase inhibitors (statins) significantly reduces risk for major ASCVD events.[6-8] Clinical trials further suggest that fibrate therapy to treat atherogenic dyslipidemia will decrease risk for ASCVD.[9,10]

Treatment of hypertension will improve prognosis for microvascular disease,[11] stroke,[12] and probably coronary heart disease. Aspirin therapy has not been shown specifically to reduce risk for ASCVD events in patients with diabetes, but its benefit for risk reduction in primary and secondary prevention in people without diabetes provides a strong rationale for using low-dose aspirin therapy in high-risk patients with type 2 diabetes. Ongoing clinical trials with antiplatelet drugs in patients with diabetes will provide more information on whether these drugs are effective in this population.

Drug Treatment of Insulin Resistance

Insulin resistance contributes to hyperglycemia, and TZDs are the major class of drugs available for treating this. Their mechanism of action is not fully understood, although their primary target of therapy seems to be peroxisome-proliferator-activated receptor (PPAR)-γ in adipose tissue, where they primarily reduce insulin resistance. In so doing, they decrease release of nonesterified fatty acids, dampen release of inflammatory cytokines and plasminogen activator inhibitor-1, and enhance adiponectin production.

The TZDs have proved useful for controlling hyperglycemia in many patients with type 2 diabetes. But they have some drawbacks that limit their use in clinical practice. They are relatively expensive, they cause edema in many patients, and precipitate congestive heart failure in some,[13] most likely secondary to fluid retention. Finally, long-term therapy is often associated with weight gain not related to fluid retention. TZDs enhance the differentiation of adipose tissue, so the availability of more adipocytes may contribute to increasing obesity. Metabolic parameters are improved despite weight gain, but it remains to be seen whether weight gain with long-term use of TZDs will have detrimental side effects that offset the benefit.

Reduction in Hepatic Glucose Output

Fasting hyperglycemia in patients with type 2 diabetes is mainly caused by increased gluconeogenesis and greater hepatic glucose output. Clinical research shows that metformin targets this pathway and reduces hepatic glucose output. The mechanism for this favorable change is not known, but the general view is that the liver is the primary target of metformin action. A few reports suggest that metformin has systemic effects that reduce insulin resistance or improve insulin secretion.[14,15]

Metformin is generally well-tolerated and has a history of generally safe long-term use in a widespread patient population. It is relatively inexpensive and tends to cause some weight reduction by curbing the appetite. One drawback is that it can cause metabolic acidosis in patients with chronic renal failure. Most physicians will not use metformin when the serum creatinine is significantly elevated. An increasing number of physicians use metformin as the first oral agent in the treatment of hyperglycemia.

Therapy to Enhance Insulin Secretion

The sulfonylureas have long been used to treat hyperglycemia of type 2 diabetes. Sulfonylureas are reported to stimulate insulin secretion by blocking ATP-sensitive potassium channels in the pancreatic β-cell membrane.[16] Because they are inexpensive, they often are used as first-line therapy. They can produce hypoglycemia, so their use must be monitored more closely than that of metformin. An alternative agent to sulfonylureas is nateglinide (Starlix®). This drug is a D-phenylalanine derivative that inhibits ATP-sensitive potassium channels in pancreatic β cells.[17] It also stimulates increased insulin secretion.

The concern that sulfonylureas could be cardiotoxic first arose in the University Group Diabetes Program (UGDP).[18] In the UGDP, treatment with the sulfonylurea tolbutamide (Orinase®) seemingly produced an increase in cardiovascular mortality. This was not confirmed in other clinical trials. The UKPDS[19] observed no indication of increased cardiovascular events or mortality with sulfonylurea treatment. In theory, the sulfonylureas might adversely affect myocardial function because their mechanism of action could impair myocardial ischemic preconditioning. Some investigators suggest that some sulfonylureas are more likely to have adverse effects on the heart than other agents.[20] The potential cardiovascular dangers of sulfonylureas are unresolved.

Combined Oral Agents

Once diabetes develops, most patients show a gradual but progressive decline in insulin secretion. This phenomenon was clearly shown in the UKPDS. In clinical practice, therapy to reduce plasma glucose levels must be progressively intensified over time to maintain acceptable control. Standard practice is to add one oral agent to another for glucose control. A common problem in clinical practice is that therapeutic regimens lag behind the decline in insulin secretion. Consequently, control of hyperglycemia declines with time. Often, insulin therapy is initiated long after it should be. This period of inadequate control can be demonstrated by the presence of hemoglobin A_{1c} levels that are well above the recommended goal.

Insulin Replacement and Therapy

Eventually, oral hypoglycemic agents will prove insufficient to maintain recommended glucose control, and insulin therapy will be required in patients with type 2 diabetes. The indications for insulin therapy must be modified by clinical judgment. However, there are some general guidelines.[21] Foremost is the need to keep plasma glucose and hemoglobin A_{1c} within recommended ranges. Most authorities agree that insulin therapy is indicated when the hemoglobin A_{1c} level cannot be maintained below 8%. Others are more aggressive in initiating insulin (ie, at hemoglobin A_{1c} levels above 7%). Glycemic control can decompensate during infection, injury, or surgery in otherwise well-controlled patients. Insulin is required in patients who exhibit progressive weight loss from glucosuria or who develop ketosis in conjunction with severe hyperglycemia. Pregnancy and renal disease often are indications for use of insulin. Patients who cannot take oral hypoglycemic agents because of side effects should receive insulin.

Hypertension

All of the clinical criteria guidelines for the metabolic syndrome include elevated blood pressure (BP) as a component. The WHO report has defined elevated BP as a metabolic syndrome component at ≥140/≥90 mm Hg. The Third Report of the Expert Panel on Detection, Evaluation, and Treatment of High Blood Cholesterol in Adults (Adult Treatment Panel III [ATP III]) and the American Association of Clinical Endocrinologists have defined elevated BP associated with the metabolic syndrome to be ≥130/≥85 mm Hg. Furthermore, a patient

Table 4-1: Blood Pressure Levels*

Classification	Systolic BP	Diastolic BP
Normal	<120	and <80
Prehypertension	120-139	or 80-89
Stage 1 hypertension	140-159	or 90-99
Stage 2 hypertension	>160	or >100

*Defined by JNC 7[22]

being treated for hypertension can be assumed to have a metabolic risk factor.

The ATP III definition of elevated BP differs slightly from that of the recently released Seventh Report of the Joint National Committee on Prevention, Detection, Evaluation, and Treatment of High Blood Pressure (JNC 7) guidelines from the National Heart, Lung, and Blood Institute.[22] JNC 7 defines two categories of hypertension and adds a third, acknowledging the linear relationship between pressure and risk of ASCVD (Table 4-1). This third category is called *prehypertension*. Eliminated from JNC 7 was a stage called *high-normal blood pressure* (SBP 130 to 139 mm Hg/DBP 85 to 89 mm Hg). ATP III identified the lower limits of high-normal BP as the threshold for elevated BP to define the metabolic syndrome.

Clinical Complications of Hypertension

Cardiovascular Disease

Hypertension is a risk factor for every form of CVD, including stroke, myocardial infarction (MI), heart failure, and chronic renal failure. Dozens of studies conclude that for individuals 40 to 70 years of age, each increment of 20 mm Hg in SBP or 10 mm Hg in DBP doubles the risk of ASCVD. This linear relationship extends across the entire BP range from 115/75 to 185/115 mm Hg.[23]

The Framingham Heart Study further demonstrated that hypertension is more likely the older one gets. Individuals with a 'normal' BP at age 55 still carry a 90% lifetime risk for developing hypertension.[24] Treatment of hypertension, conversely, lowers risk for its complications. Antihypertensive therapy produces reductions in stroke incidence averaging 35% to 40%; MI, 20% to 25%; and heart failure, more than 50%.[25]

Proteinuria

Proteinuria is considered a metabolic dysfunction of renal glomeruli related to hypertension. Its presence carries predictive power for CVD events. This is true in hypertensive patients with and without diabetes.

Association of Hypertension With Type 2 Diabetes

Hypertension is strongly associated with type 2 diabetes and proportionally related to cardiovascular mortality in diabetic patients. When other components of the metabolic syndrome are added to hypertension, the risk is substantially increased. This linear increase demonstrates dramatically the intimate interrelationship among all the components, because which components are present appears to matter less than the combined synergistic influence of each additional one.

Benefits of Hypertension Treatment

JNC 7 reviewed benefits from treatment of hypertension as revealed by a large number of clinical trials.[22] For patients who have stage 1 hypertension (SBP 140 to 159 mm Hg and/or DBP 90 to 99 mm Hg) plus other CVD risk factors, achieving a sustained 12 mm Hg reduction in SBP over 10 years will prevent one death for every 11 patients treated. When CVD or target organ damage is present, only nine patients will require such BP reduction to prevent one death.[26]

The Systolic Hypertension in Europe (Syst-Eur) study and the Hypertension Optimal Treatment (HOT) Study Group both found benefits from controlling BP in type 2 diabetes.[27] Compared to placebo, active treatment produced a 41% drop in overall mortality, a 70% drop in cardiovascular mortality, a 62% drop in all cardiovascular events, a 69% drop in stroke, and a 57% drop in all cardiac events. The HOT study found the greatest benefit to occur at a DBP <80 mm Hg.[28] Syst-Eur studied nitrendipine vs placebo in 492 diabetic patients; HOT evaluated the difference between treating a DBP of 90 mm Hg vs 80 mm Hg using felodipine (Plendil®).

Among the many trials that proved the effectiveness of angiotensin-converting enzyme (ACE) inhibitors, the Heart Outcomes Prevention Evaluation Study (HOPE) trial[29] studied the effect of ramipril (Altace®) in 3,577 diabetic patients with at least one cardiovascular risk factor but no proteinuria and no heart failure. The cardiovascular benefit was greater than that attributable to the decrease in BP. The investigators concluded that ACE inhibitors yield a vasculoprotective and renoprotective effect for people with diabetes. ACE inhibitors proved efficacious in three other trials:

- Captopril (Capoten®) was compared with placebo in 207 insulin-dependent (type 1) diabetics with proteinuria. Captopril treatment was associated with a 50% reduction in the risk of the combined end points of death, dialysis, and transplantation. The addition of a diuretic was required to control BP in 75% of patients.[30]
- 583 patients with renal insufficiency caused by various disorders were treated with benazepril (Lotensin®) for 3 years. The primary end point was a doubling of the baseline serum creatine concentration or the need for dialysis. Benazepril reduced the risk of reaching these points by 53%.[31]
- In a 7-year study of 94 type 2 diabetics with normal BP and microalbuminuria, treatment with enalapril (Vasotec®) resulted in an absolute risk reduction of 42% for nephropathy.[32]

The Losartan Intervention for Endpoint (LIFE) study compared losartan (Cozaar®, Hyzaar®) with atenolol (Tenormin®) in more than 9,000 patients and in a subgroup of 1,195 patients with diabetes. The relative risk for the primary end point—a primary cardiovascular event (death, MI, or stroke)—favored losartan with a risk ratio of 0.87. For the diabetic subset, the risk ratio was even more favorable to losartan—0.76. The all-cause mortality also favored losartan, with a risk ratio in the diabetic subgroup of 0.61 ($P = 0.002$).[33,34]

The Fosinopril Versus Amlodipine Cardiovascular Events Randomized Trial (FACET) included 380 Italian patients with hypertension and type 2 diabetes. Fosinopril (Monopril®) and amlodipine (Norvasc®) had similar effects on biochemical measures (cholesterol, high-density lipoprotein [HDL] cholesterol, glycosylated hemoglobin, fasting serum glucose, and plasma insulin), but, compared with patients receiving amlodipine, patients receiving fosinopril had a significantly lower risk of the combined outcome of acute MI, stroke, or hospitalized angina (14/189 vs 27/191; hazards ratio = 0.49).[35]

The Appropriate Blood Pressure Control in Diabetes (ABCD) study followed 470 hypertensive, type 2 diabetic patients without overt albuminuria on nisoldipine (Sular®) or enalapril for 5.3 years to compare the effect of intensive and less-intensive BP control on the microvascular complications of diabetes. The intensively treated group achieved an average BP of 132/78 mm Hg; the other group averaged 138/86 mm Hg. There was no difference between the two drugs or the two BP goals in stabilization of renal function.

The Captopril Prevention Project (CAPPP) studied 10,985 patients from Sweden and Finland to compare ACE inhibition with conventional therapy in preventing fatal and nonfatal MI, stroke, and other cardiovascular deaths in patients with hypertension. Cardiovascular mortality was lower with captopril than with conventional treatment (76 vs 95 events; relative risk 0.77, $P = 0.092$), but fatal and nonfatal stroke was more common with captopril (189 vs 148; relative risk 1.25; $P = 0.044$).[36]

These three studies—ABCD, FACET, and CAPPP—demonstrated the superiority of ACE inhibitors over alternative treatments in reducing the risk of acute MI (63% reduction, P <0.001), cardiovascular events (51% reduction, P <0.001), and all-cause mortality (62% reduction, P = 0.010). In none of the trials did the ACE inhibitors demonstrate any advantage in preventing stroke.[37]

The Prospective Randomized Amlodipine Survival Evaluation (PRAISE)[38] followed 1,153 patients with NYHA class IIIb or IV heart failure for a median 14.5 months on amlodipine (a long-lasting dihydropyridine [DHP] calcium channel blocker [CCB]) or placebo. All patients were also taking ACE inhibitors, diuretics, and digitalis. The investigators concluded that amlodipine reduced pump failure and sudden deaths only in nonischemic heart failure patients. Ischemic heart failure did not benefit from amlodipine.

The African American Study of Kidney Disease and Hypertension (AASK) compared ramipril, an ACE inhibitor, with amlodipine, a DHP CCB, in African-American patients with hypertension and renal insufficiency. Three years into the study, the ramipril group experienced sufficiently less decline in renal function to end the study. The authors recommended that DHP CCBs be used with caution in patients with renal insufficiency.[39]

Taken together, studies of diabetic patients with hypertension demonstrate a benefit over and above that seen in patients without diabetes. Moreover, the benefit extends well into what was considered a 'normal' range of BP readings.

Pharmacologic Treatment of Elevated Blood Pressure

Trials of BP treatment have tested every hypertensive agent and nearly every combination available. A common finding of all trials is the need to use more than one drug. As Figure 4-1 shows, an average of three agents was used in the six studies.

Thiazides and Potassium Sparers

Thiazide diuretics have been the foundation of nearly every antihypertensive regimen. Nevertheless, diuretics are

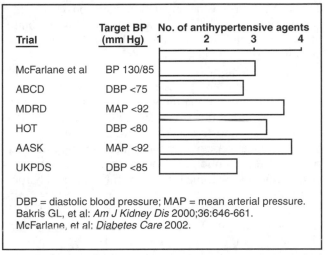

DBP = diastolic blood pressure; MAP = mean arterial pressure.
Bakris GL, et al: *Am J Kidney Dis* 2000;36:646-661.
McFarlane, et al: *Diabetes Care* 2002.

Figure 4-1: Multiple antihypertensive agents needed to achieve target blood pressure in different trials.

still underused in practice,[40] for two reasons. First, other medications are more heavily promoted by pharmaceutical companies. Second, concerns exist about the adverse effects of thiazides on lipids, glucose levels, and electrolytes.

Higher doses of thiazides raise triglyceride levels[41] and decrease insulin sensitivity.[42,43] The decrease in insulin sensitivity, probably mediated by hypokalemia,[44] has been nullified by adding potassium-sparing diuretics and has been shown to be of minor significance when lower doses are used (eg, 12.5 mg q.d. of hydrochlorothiazide [Dyazide®]).[40,44] The clinical significance of these effects is questionable in view of the substantial success thiazides have had in reducing end point events, even in patients who experience elevated lipid and glucose levels, especially when low doses are used.[45,46] Using thiazides as treatment for hypertension may generate excessive complications from diabetes later. JNC 7 still recommends thiazides as first-line therapy for hypertension. However, it is prudent to keep the dose relatively low and to monitor potassium levels, although it is unclear if potassium sparing will help avoid diabetes complications.

Spironolactone (Aldactone®) has been reported to promote magnesium and potassium retention, increase uptake of myocardial norepinephrine, and attenuate formation of myocardial fibrosis. These effects are the result of counteracting aldosterone's inhibition of catecholamine reuptake, enhancement of potassium and magnesium excretion, and promotion of ventricular arrhythmias, myocardial fibrosis, endothelial cell dysfunction, and baroreceptor dysfunction.[47]

A recently released alternative to spironolactone is eplerenone (Inspra™), which has shown efficacy when given as an adjunct to angiotensin II receptor blocker (ARB) therapy and has proved its usefulness in heart failure in the Eplerenone Post-MI Heart Failure Efficacy and Survival Study (EPHESUS), causing fewer side effects (especially in men) than spironolactone.[48]

Renin-Angiotensin-Aldosterone System Blockade

Among the multiple classes of agents available for treating hypertension, ACE inhibitors and ARBs uniquely slow the progress of diabetic nephropathy and reduce albuminuria.[30,49,50] The Reduction of Endpoints in NIDDM with the Angiotensin II Antagonist Losartan (RENAAL) trial has shown that treatment with losartan substantially reduces the incidence of end-stage renal disease.[51] Additionally, ACE inhibitors, when combined with diuretics, have proved their value by increasing survival in patients with left-ventricular systolic failure, with an average risk reduction of 35% for the combined end points of mortality and hospitalization for heart failure.[52]

The choice between ACE inhibitors and ARBs depends on cost and the physician's greater experience with ACE inhibitors. ARBs are recommended primarily for patients who do not tolerate ACE inhibitors, usually because of the dry cough that is a common side effect. Theoretic differences exist between the two classes of agents. ACE inhibitors prevent the conversion of angiotensin to an active form, while ARBs allow angiotensin to be activated but prevent it from acting on specific target tissues. This may become important because angiotensin has effects that are not blocked by ARBs and generation pathways that bypass angiotensinogen conversion. Further research will uncover these effects and their clinical significance, if any.

The Valsartan Heart Failure Trial (Val-Heft) has warned of an antagonistic effect when ACE inhibitors and ARBs are used together. When added to prescribed therapy, valsartan (Diovan®) significantly reduces the combined end point of mortality and morbidity and improves clinical signs and symptoms in patients with heart failure. But patients taking valsartan and an ACE inhibitor did substantially worse than those taking valsartan alone. Those taking both experienced a 2.1% reduction in adverse cardiac events compared with those taking valsartan alone, who reduced their events by 13.1% (both results compared with placebo).[53] Further meta-analyses of several clinical trials that included the combination of an ACE inhibitor with an ARB have reached different conclusions. One[54,55] concluded that an ARB combined with an ACE inhibitor may benefit heart failure patients who are receiving all other recommended therapies, while another[56] limited its recommendation to patients not on β-blockers.

Another issue about modulating the renin-angiotensin-aldosterone system (RAAS) is its potential to delay the onset of type 2 diabetes. One review[57] tentatively concluded that data from the highest quality studies suggest that diabetes incidence is unchanged or increased by thiazide diuretics and β-blockers and unchanged or decreased by ACE inhibitors, CCBs, and ARBs.

α_1-Blockers

The α_1-blockers include doxazosin (Cardura®), prazosin (Minipress®), and terazosin (Hytrin®). α_1-Blockers improve insulin sensitivity and dyslipidemia[58]; however, they seem to be less effective than other antihypertensive agents in reducing cardiovascular events. In the ALLHAT study,[59] doxazosin exhibited a higher incidence of stroke, heart failure, and combined cardiovascular events compared to a thiazide. The use of α_1-blockers has largely been relegated to second or third choices.

β-Blockers Without β$_2$-Agonism

Many β-blockers are not β$_2$-agonists. These agents include atenolol, betaxolol (Kerlone®), bisoprolol (Zebeta®), metoprolol (Lopressor®), extended-release metoprolol (Toprol XL®), nadolol (Corgard®), propranolol (Inderal®), long-acting propranolol (Inderal® LA), and timolol (Blocadren®) and can be divided into selective β$_1$-blockers and nonselective β$_1$- and β$_2$-blockers. Among the former, atenolol and metoprolol are the most widely used and are considered preferable because they induce less bronchial constriction and vasoconstriction. β$_1$ Blockade slows the heart rate, weakens heart contractions, and decreases RAAS activity.[60]

β-Blockers have been proven to reduce MI and stroke. They are inexpensive, available as generics, and come in once-daily dose formulations (atenolol and extended-release metoprolol). JNC 7 recommends them as first-line treatment for patients without diabetes who have hypertension or previous coronary syndromes.[22] They carry a variety of side effects: fatigue, sexual dysfunction, cold extremities, depression, weight gain, negative inotropy and chronotropy, and asthma. Additionally, the suppressive effects of β-blockers on cardiac function may threaten an already marginal blood supply to other organs in patients with peripheral vascular disease.

The β$_1$-selective blocking agents, such as metoprolol and atenolol, have been reported to produce increased insulin resistance associated with increased fasting values of insulin and glucose. They may also suppress insulin secretion. These changes are associated with some increase in serum triglycerides and decreases in HDL cholesterol. Consequently, in theory, β_1-selective β-blockers are not desirable agents to use in patients with the metabolic syndrome.

Of concern for patients with the metabolic syndrome is the action of β-blockers to increase insulin resistance and to mask the BP changes and tachycardia that announce an episode of hypoglycemia, a fairly rare event in type 2 diabetes. However, other symptoms of hypoglycemia, such as dizziness and sweating, still occur.[61] Despite concern about the use of β-blockers in patients with diabetes, the UKPDS demonstrated that a β-blocker was just as effective as an ACE inhibitor in reducing microvascular disease in patients with type 2 diabetes.[62]

β-Blockers With β_2-Agonism

β_2-Agonist β-blockers include acebutolol (Sectral®), penbutolol (Levatol®), and pindolol (Visken®). These agents are nonselective β-adrenergic blockers that have partial agonist action at vascular β_2 receptors. They have been approved for the treatment of systemic hypertension. They have fewer adverse effects on glucose tolerance and serum lipoprotein profile than β-blockers without sympathomimetic activity. Because of the more favorable metabolic effects of these agents compared to β_1-selective β-blockers, they should be more desirable for use in treatment of hypertension in patients with the metabolic syndrome.

β-Blockers With α_1 Blockade

This class contains carvedilol (Coreg®) and labetalol (Normodyne®, Trandate®). Carvedilol has apparent benefit in the treatment of congestive heart failure. It is a nonselective β-adrenoreceptor antagonist combined with an α_1-adrenoreceptor antagonist. It is devoid of intrinsic sympathomimetic activity. Studies have shown that carvedilol causes fewer negative chronotropic and inotropic effects when compared with other nonselective β-blockers such as propranolol. Because it is a peripheral vasodilator, it seemingly improves renal blood flow more

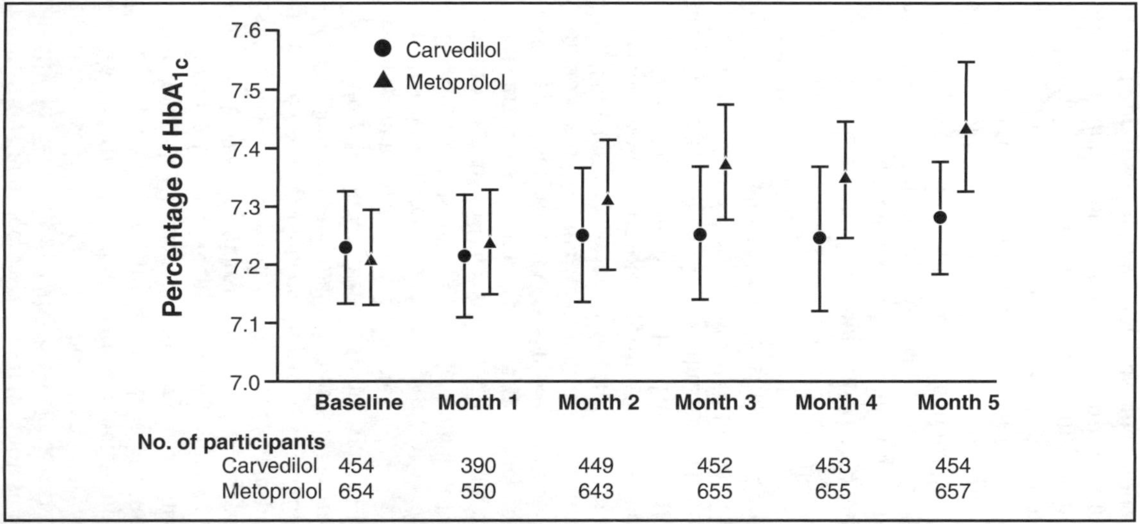

Figure 4-2: Glycosylated hemoglobin A_{1c} at baseline and each maintenance month by treatment in the modified intention-to-treat population. The change from baseline to maintenance month 5 (primary outcome) was significant (mean difference [SD], 0.13% [0.05%]; 95% confidence interval, -0.22% to -0.04%; P=.004). Error bars indicate SD from mean. Bakris et al,[63] used with permission.

than nonselective β-blockers. Carvedilol may have other beneficial effects such as calcium channel blocking and antioxidant properties.

One potential advantage of carvedilol over other non-selective and selective β-blockers is that it appears to have fewer adverse metabolic effects. The metabolic changes of carvedilol were compared to those of metoprolol in the Glycemic Effects in Diabetes Mellitus: Carvedilol-Metoprolol Comparison in Hypertensives (GEMINI) study.[63] GEMINI was designed to study patients with diabetes and hypertension who were already being treated with an ACE inhibitor or an ARB and whose blood pressure was not controlled. If needed for BP control, open-label hydrochlorothiazide and a dihydropyridine calcium antagonist were allowed in the study. Both carvedilol and metoprolol were given in divided doses daily and were added to ACE inhibitor or ARB therapy. The primary end point of the study was the difference between groups and mean change from baseline hemoglobin A_{1c}. Other measures included the effects of the two drugs on fasting insulin levels, HOMA-IR, BP, and plasma lipids. Throughout the trial, carvedilol and metoprolol were well tolerated.

The changes in hemoglobin A_{1c} longitudinally throughout the study are shown in Figure 4-2.[63] Other metabolic changes generally were more favorable on carvedilol than on metoprolol[64] (Table 4-2). BP changes were similar for the two drugs. Insulin resistance was significantly improved on carvedilol compared to metoprolol.[63] Moreover, progression to microalbuminuria with carvedilol was reduced to 47% of that with metoprolol.[63]

Carvedilol did not worsen metabolic control in patients with type 2 diabetes, but a worsening was observed for those treated with metoprolol.[63] This study has implications for treatment of patients with the metabolic syndrome. In patients with impaired fasting glucose or impaired glucose tolerance, the use of usual β-blockers such as metoprolol can cause a worsening of glucose

Table 4-2: Cardiovascular and Metabolic Measures in the GEMINI Study*

Parameter	Carvedilol (n = 454) % Change	Metoprolol (n = 657) % Change
Systolic blood pressure	-17.9 (0.7)	-16.9
Diastolic blood pressure	-10.0 (0.4)	-10.3
Mean heart rate	-6.7 (0.4)	- 8.3
ACR**	-14.0	+2.5
HOMA-IR†	-9.1	-2.0
Plasma glucose	+6.6	+10.6
Serum albumin	-19.4	-15.1
Body weight	+0.17	+1.2
Total cholesterol	-3.3	-0.4
LDL cholesterol	-4.4	-2.7
HDL cholesterol	-5.5	-5.7
Triglycerides	+2.2	+13.2

*Modified intention-to-treat analysis
**Urinary albumin/creatinine ratio
†Homeostatic Model Assessment—Insulin Resistance
Adapted from Bakris et al,[63] used with permission.

tolerance, causing some patients to cross the glycemic threshold for type 2 diabetes. In addition, for patients with type 2 diabetes, metoprolol and related agents can cause a worsening of glycemic control. The fact that carvedilol does not have this adverse effect appears to be a distinct advantage for treatment of hypertension in patients with the metabolic syndrome and with (Table 4-3) or without type 2 diabetes.[63]

Calcium Channel Blockers

Calcium channel blockers (CCBs) are commonly used because of their dual indications (hypertension and angina) and their low cost. CCBs, along with diuretics, appear to be more efficacious in African Americans, whose generally more severe hypertension responds less to monotherapy with β-blockers, ACE inhibitors, or ARBs. Combination therapy, as well as adequate diuresis, overcomes this discrepancy, but ACE inhibitor-induced angioedema occurs 2 to 4 times more frequently in African Americans.[65]

The primary difference between the two types of CCBs—nondihydropyridines (verapamil [Calan®] and diltiazem [Cardizem®]) and dihydropyridines (all the rest)—is their effect on cardiac conduction. The nondihydropyridines slow cardiac conduction and are more likely to cause serious arrhythmias. There are also major differences in the pharmacokinetics among the dozen-or-so agents available. Short-acting agents such as nifedipine (Procardia®) have been reported to increase the incidence of coronary events.[66,67] Longer-lasting agents such as amlodipine therefore are recommended for treating hypertension.

Combination Therapies

A combination agent has been introduced for the metabolic syndrome that addresses two of its components in a single pill. Amlodipine, a CCB, and atorvastatin, an HMG CoA reductase inhibitor, are available together in eight different strengths (Caduet®). Several studies have suggested efficacy of this combination, such as in improving nitric oxide release and endothelial function,[68] retarding progression of coronary atherosclerosis,[69] and improving arterial compliance.[70]

Table 4-3: Considerations for Choice of Antihypertensive Drugs in Patients With the Metabolic Syndrome and Type 2 Diabetes

Agent	Comments
Thiazide diuretics	• Inexpensive; JNC 7 first-line drug • Increased diabetes incidence in ALLHAT • Glucose intolerance worsened by hypokalemia
Potassium-sparing diuretics	• May reduce incidence of hypokalemia with thiazides • Can induce hyperkalemia with angiotensin-converting enzyme (ACE) inhibitors in patients with diabetes
β-Blockers ($\beta_1 \pm \beta_2$ blockers)	• Can worsen glucose intolerance in patients with impaired fasting glucose/impaired glucose tolerance or type 2 diabetes • Can raise serum triglycerides and reduce high-density lipoprotein • Reduce microvascular end points similarly to ACE inhibitor in UKPDS patients
β-Blockers with sympathomimetic activity (β_1, β_2 blocker + β_2 agonist)	• Less worsening of glucose tolerance and fewer adverse effects on lipid profiles compared to β-blockers without sympathomimetic activity

ALLHAT = Antihypertensive and Lipid-Lowering Treatment to Prevent Heart Attack Trial

Agent	Comments
Combined α- and β-blockers ($\beta_1 \pm \beta_2$ blockers + α_1-blocker)	• No adverse effect on glucose tolerance or serum lipoprotein profile • Metabolically superior to pure β-blockers (GEMINI)
ACE inhibitors and angiotensin receptor blockers	• No adverse effect on glucose tolerance or serum lipoprotein profile • Improve clinical outcomes in patients with chronic renal failure (with or without diabetes) • May be superior to other antihypertensive agents in secondary prevention to reduce atherosclerotic cardiovascular disease events
Calcium blockers	• No adverse metabolic effects
α_1-Blockers	• Improves glucose and lipid profiles • Less effective on stroke, heart failure, and cardiovascular disease outcomes than thiazide diuretics (ALLHAT)

GEMINI = Glycemic Effects in Diabetes Mellitus: Carvedilol-Metoprolol Comparison in Hypertensives, JNC 7 = Seventh Report of the Joint National Committee on Prevention, Detection, Evaluation, and Treatment of High Blood Pressure, UKPDS = United Kingdom Prospective Diabetes Study

Atherogenic Dyslipidemia

Atherogenic dyslipidemia consists of the following lipid abnormalities in the serum:

- elevations of apolipoprotein B (apo B)
- elevations of triglyceride-rich lipoproteins (TGRLP)
- elevations of small low-density lipoprotein (LDL) particles
- low high-density lipoprotein (HDL) cholesterol.

All of these abnormalities enhance the risk for atherosclerotic cardiovascular disease (ASCVD). Thus, management of atherogenic dyslipidemia is critical for the appropriate management of cardiovascular disease. First-line treatment of atherogenic dyslipidemia is therapeutic lifestyle changes (TLC); however, if abnormalities persist after lifestyle therapies, drug therapy may be required.

Goals of Lipid-lowering Therapy

Elevations of Apolipoprotein B-containing Lipoproteins

There are three potential targets of therapy among the apo B-containing lipoproteins: LDL cholesterol, very low-density lipoprotein (VLDL) + LDL (non-HDL) cholesterol, and total apo B. ATP III defines goals of therapy according to a patient's risk status for coronary heart disease (CHD).[71] In those with isolated elevations of LDL, serum LDL cholesterol is a sufficient target of treatment. However, in those with other components of atherogenic dyslipidemia, as is typical of the metabolic syndrome, the other components should be included in therapy. According to ATP III, even in patients with the metabolic syndrome, LDL cholesterol remains the primary target of therapy. However, when atherogenic dyslipidemia is identified, usually by elevation of triglyceride (TG) levels, VLDL+LDL cholesterol becomes a secondary target. The total apo B can be used as an alternative to VLDL+LDL cholesterol. Table 4-4 shows suggested goals of treatment for different categories of risk.

Elevated Triglyceride Levels

According to ATP III, when TG is elevated, non-HDL cholesterol levels (or total apo B) become secondary targets of therapy. In ATP III, the TG cut point for adding these secondary treatment targets is 200 mg/dL. However, it is reasonable to introduce these measures as secondary targets when people have TG levels >150 mg/dL plus the metabolic syndrome. Triglycerides become a direct target of lipid-lowering therapy only when levels exceed 500 mg/dL. When TG levels are very high, the risk for acute pancreatitis increases. Triglyceride-lowering therapy must then be introduced. The goal is to reduce TG levels to <500 mg/dL, a level that will not cause pancreatitis. When TG is in the range of 150 to 499 mg/dL, VLDL remnants represent a risk factor. However, elevations of remnant lipoproteins are identified in the non-HDL cholesterol fraction. Therefore, therapies for TG in this range are better directed against non-HDL cholesterol (or total apo B) rather than against elevated TG.

Small LDL Particles

Although small LDL particles probably introduce added risk to the metabolic syndrome, they generally do not represent unique targets of therapy, according to ATP III. Elevations of small LDL particles contribute to higher levels of non-HDL cholesterol and total apo B. Thus, they are included among all of the apo B-containing lipoproteins that are the secondary targets of treatment. In short, LDL cholesterol is the primary target of therapy, and non-HDL cholesterol (including total apo B and small LDL particles) is a secondary target. There are two ways that small LDL particles can be changed to reduce CHD risk: reducing their number or converting them to larger LDL. Therapies reducing TG levels usually lead to a conversion of smaller to larger LDL.[72]

Low HDL Levels

ATP III identifies a low HDL-cholesterol level as a tertiary target of treatment, after LDL cholesterol and non-HDL cholesterol. Although low HDL-cholesterol levels are highly predictive of risk for CVD, there is little clini-

Table 4-4: Treatment Goals for LDL Cholesterol, non-HDL Cholesterol, and Total Apo B

Risk Status	Primary Target: LDL Cholesterol Therapeutic Goal (mg/dL)
High risk Very high risk	<100 mg/dL (optional <70 mg/dL)
Moderately high risk (2+ risk factors* and 10-year risk 10% to 20%)	<130 mg/dL (optional: <100 mg/dL)
Moderate risk (2+ risk factors and 10-year risk <10%)	<130 mg/dL
Lower risk (0-1 risk factor)	<160 mg/dL

* Risk factors include cigarette smoking, hypertension (blood pressure >140/90 mm Hg or on antihypertensive medication), low HDL cholesterol (<40 mg/dL), family history of premature CHD (CHD in first-degree male relative <55 years; CHD in first-degree female relative <65 years), and age (men >45 years; women >55 years).

cal trial evidence that therapies directed toward raising HDL cholesterol reduce risk. For this reason, ATP III does not specify a particular goal for HDL. Although increasing HDL levels may protect against atherosclerosis, the evidence is scant to make specific recommen-

Secondary Target: non-HDL Cholesterol** Therapeutic Goal (mg/dL)	Secondary Target: Total Apo B*** Therapeutic Goal (mg/dL)
<130 mg/dL (optional <100 mg/dL)	<90 mg/dL
<160 mg/dL (optional: <130 mg/dL)	<110 mg/dL
<160 mg/dL	<110 mg/dL
<190 mg/dL	<130 mg/dL

** non-HDL cholesterol becomes a secondary goal of therapy when serum TG levels range from 200 to 500 mg/dL. It is calculated as total cholesterol minus HDL.

*** Apo B is an alternative secondary goal of therapy when serum TG levels range from 200 to 500 mg/dL.

dations. However, the pharmaceutical industry is heavily engaged in efforts to develop new and more effective HDL-raising drugs. If such drugs can be shown to reduce risk, they undoubtedly would find a place in the treatment of atherogenic dyslipidemia.

Drug Therapies for Atherogenic Dyslipidemia

The hydroxymethyl glutaryl coenzyme A (HMG CoA) reductase inhibitors (statins) are highly effective drugs for reducing apo B-containing lipoproteins. They primarily lower LDL levels but also lower atherogenic remnant lipoproteins. Numerous clinical trials document the efficacy of statins for reducing risk in higher-risk patients.[71] No single trial has exclusively tested patients with the metabolic syndrome, but subgroup analysis of the major statin trials strongly suggests that these drugs reduce risk for CVD in these patients.[73] Statins have proved generally safe in clinical practice. Six statins are available in clinical practice; these are listed in Table 4-5 along with standard doses and average LDL-cholesterol reductions. One other statin, cerivastatin, was removed from the market because it proved to have a side effect/efficacy ratio that was too high to sustain its use in clinical practice.

Statins lower apo B-containing lipoproteins by increasing hepatic expression of LDL receptors. Normally, statins act almost exclusively in the liver. They reduce the synthesis of cholesterol by inhibiting hepatic HMG CoA reductase.[74,75] This action lowers the cholesterol content of liver cells, which in turn increases the synthesis of LDL receptors. LDL receptors interact with circulating lipoproteins containing apo B. They mediate the removal of these lipoproteins (LDL and VLDL remnants) from the circulation. Statins given in high doses may also reduce the secretion of lipoproteins by the liver.

The dose-response relationship between statin dose and LDL lowering is not proportional. Generally, for every doubling of the dose of statins, LDL cholesterol concentrations fall by another 6%. Thus, tripling the dose lowers LDL-cholesterol levels by about 12%, and quadrupling the dose, by 18%. However, the dose of statin required to produce various reductions of LDL varies. A standard dose of statin is one that produces a 30% to 40% reduction of LDL cholesterol.

Table 4-5: LDL-Cholesterol Average Reduction With Standard Doses of Available Statins

Drug	Dose (mg/d)	LDL reduction (%)
Atorvastatin (Lipitor®)	10	39
Fluvastatin (Lescol®)	40-80	25-31
Lovastatin (Mevacor®)	40	31
Nicotinic acid/lovastatin (Advicor®)	1,000/40	36
Pravastatin (Pravachol®)	40	34
Rosuvastatin (Crestor®)	5-10	39-45
Simvastatin (Zocor®)	20-40	35-41

Major clinical trials with statin therapy have reported a reduction in ASCVD.[71] Disease reductions include acute coronary syndromes (unstable angina, myocardial infarction, and coronary death), coronary procedures, various other coronary outcomes, and stroke. Statin therapy reduces new-onset and recurrent CVD events. Because of these trials, statins have emerged as first-line cholesterol-lowering therapy.

Three primary prevention trials of statin therapy are the West of Scotland Coronary Prevention Study (WOSCOPS),[76] the Air Force/Texas Coronary Atherosclerosis Prevention Study (AFCAPS/TexCAPS),[77] and the Anglo-Scandinavian Cardiac Outcomes Trial—Lipid Lowering Arm (ASCOT-LLA).[78] In all three trials, statin treatment significantly reduced relative risk (RR) for major coronary events. In WOSCOPS, a strong trend toward a decrease in total mortality was observed. In AFCAPS/ TexCAPS and ASCOT, the number of deaths was too small to draw any conclusions about effects of statin therapy on total mortality. Nonetheless, no increase in noncardiovascular mortality was observed. In fact, even nonfatal adverse effects were rare.

Similar reductions in RR for ASCVD events were obtained in high-risk patients in secondary prevention trials. However, there was a greater benefit for higher-risk patients because of their higher absolute risk. New trials published since publication of ATP III are the Heart Protection Study (HPS)[79] and the Prospective Study of Pravastatin in the Elderly at Risk (PROSPER).[80] In these trials, statin therapy was efficacious for all types of patients. Similar reductions in RR were observed for men vs women, older vs younger patients, smokers vs nonsmokers, hypertensives vs normotensives, and patients with diabetes vs those without.

Statins are not entirely free of side effects. Occasionally, patients will have gastrointestinal (GI) complaints or will manifest skin or allergic reactions. Insomnia has been reported but has been difficult to verify in specific studies. The same is true for nonspecific weakness and myalgia. Some patients respond to statin therapy, particularly at higher doses, with elevations of hepatic transaminases. The major concern, although rare, is myopathy.[81]

The clinical significance of elevated serum transaminases is uncertain. The major concern, of course, is hepatotoxicity. That statins cause liver injury by predisposing people to cirrhosis or chronic liver disease is doubtful; there is no documentation. Some authorities believe that modest rises in transaminases are a physiologic response to the drug and do not indicate true hepatotoxicity. Routine monitoring of liver function tests for patients on statin therapy seems to be unnecessary.

However, statins can definitely cause myopathy. Complaints of myalgia with statin therapy are relatively common. Although many patients and physicians believe in statin-induced myalgias, clinical trials have not verified their existence. The frequencies of such complaints in placebo and statin-treated groups are similar. In clinical practice, physicians should take a patient's complaints seriously and work through them with the goal of maintaining statin therapy. Frequently, the complaint can be shown to relate to another condition (eg, arthritis, tendonitis). Switching to another statin sometimes eliminates the complaint, as does lowering the dose.

The development of moderate but persistent elevations of creatine kinase (CK) requires attention. If these elevations can be shown to be caused by statin treatment, the drug may need to be discontinued. Nonetheless, it must be remembered that other causes elevate CK (eg, other muscle disease, mild forms of trauma). African Americans often normally exhibit what would be considered moderate elevations in whites. Finally, the procedures listed above for myalgias can be tried in patients with moderate CK elevations with the aim of maintaining effective therapy.

Severe myopathy is the most feared side effect of statin therapy. It is characterized by muscle pain and weakness, CK elevations >10 times normal, and brown urine (myoglobinuria). The latter can cause acute renal failure, which may result in death. An unacceptably high frequency of severe myopathy and renal failure led to the removal of cerivastatin from the market. Certain risk factors predict the development of severe myopathy (Table 4-6).[81]

For patients with the metabolic syndrome, the combination of statin + gemfibrozil (Lopid®) significantly increases risk for myopathy. This risk is much lower when a statin is combined with fenofibrate (TriCor®, Lofibra™). However, when this combination is used, avoid high doses of statins. Generally, statin therapy should be avoided or doses kept low in patients who have risk factors for statin-induced myopathy.

Table 4-6: Risk Factors for Severe Myopathy

- Older people who are frail or have a small body frame, especially older women

- Presence of multisystem disease (especially debilitated status)

- Chronic renal insufficiency (including diabetic renal disease)

- Chronic liver disease

- Hypothyroidism

- Coadministration of multiple medications, particularly gemfibrozil, cyclosporine, azole antifungals (itraconazole and ketoconazole), macrolide antibiotics (erythromycin and clarithromycin), HIV protease inhibitors, the antidepressant nefazodone, and verapamil.

- Severe illnesses and perioperative periods. Statins should usually be withheld when patients are admitted to the hospital for acute illnesses or for major surgery.

- Alcohol abuse

- Heavy exercise

- Daily consumption of large quantities of grapefruit juice (eg >1 quart per day)

Add-on LDL-lowering Drugs to Statin Therapy

Although statins represent primary therapy for reducing LDL, VLDL+LDL, and apo B, standard doses often fail to achieve the goals of therapy outlined in Table 4-4. One approach to attaining the therapeutic goal is to increase the dose of the statin. For every doubling of the statin dose, the LDL-cholesterol level will be reduced by approximately 6%. In uncomplicated individuals, high doses of statins are usually well tolerated, and the goals of therapy are often achieved. However, in people who carry risk factors for severe myopathy, the standard dose of statin usually should not be exceeded. This includes the concomitant use of fibrates such as fenofibrate. In such cases, the goals of therapy may better be attained by using LDL-lowering drugs in combination. Among the latter, the cholesterol-absorption blockers and the bile acid absorption blockers are most frequently used.

Cholesterol-absorption Blockers

One category of cholesterol-absorption blockers is the plant stanols and sterols. These are naturally occurring sterols found in plants and incorporated into two margarines (Benecol® and Take Control®). In a dose of about 2 g/d, they will reduce LDL-cholesterol levels by 10% to 15%[82,83] and enhance the LDL reduction achieved by dietary means. They further reduce LDL-cholesterol levels in individuals taking statins.

Another cholesterol-absorption blocker is ezetimibe (Zetia®),[84,85] which typically lowers LDL-cholesterol levels by 15% to 22%. The drug appears to be safe, with no serious side effects reported. When ezetimibe is combined with standard doses of statins, an additional 15% to 22% reduction in LDL-cholesterol levels can be obtained. This equates to a quadrupling of the statin dose.

Bile Acid Absorption Blockers

Bile acid absorption blockers bind to bile acids in the intestine and thus prevent reabsorption. Blocking return of bile acids to the liver releases feedback inhibition, promoting conversion of cholesterol to bile acids in the liver. Thus, more cholesterol is converted into bile acids, and hepatic cholesterol concentrations fall. This stimulates the synthesis of LDL receptors, which in turn lowers serum LDL levels. Depending on the dose of bile acid absorption blocker, the LDL level can be reduced by 15% to 30%.

When moderate doses of these agents are added to statin therapy, the LDL level usually falls by an additional 15% to 20%, equivalent to quadrupling the dose of statin.[86]

Three bile acid absorption blockers are available for therapy: cholestyramine (Prevalite®), colestipol (Colestid®), and colesevelam (Welchol®). Moderate doses of the first two are 8 and 10 g/d, respectively. Colesevelam is a new bile acid absorption blocker that is effective for LDL reduction in lower doses than similar agents.[87] The usual dose of colesevelam is 3.75 g/d.

Bile acid absorption blockers act exclusively in the GI tract, where they can produce upper GI distress or constipation, both of which usually abate with continued use. Constipation can usually be prevented by taking a psyllium-based bulking agent. Early research suggested that bile acid absorption blockers also could block the absorption of other drugs (eg, digoxin, warfarin, thyroxine, thiazide diuretics, β-blockers). Therefore, these agents should not be administered simultaneously with the blocker. Bile acid absorption blockers can raise TG levels, so they should be avoided in patients with severe hypertriglyceridemia. They can, however, be used in patients with mild elevations of TG, such as those with type 2 diabetes.[88]

Drugs That Primarily Reduce Triglyceride-rich Lipoproteins and Raise HDL Cholesterol
Fibric acid derivatives (fibrates)
Although fibrates were once considered useful only for severe hypertriglyceridemia, their use has been increasing.

The three fibrates available in the United States are clofibrate (Atromid-S®), gemfibrozil, and fenofibrate. Clofibrate is rarely used anymore. Other fibrates with similar actions are available, however. Although gemfibrozil has been the most widely used fibrate in the United States, use of fenofibrate is growing. Fenofibrate seemingly has the advantage of safety when used in combination with a statin, which makes it an attractive choice for patients with the metabolic syndrome.

Effects of fibrates on lipid and lipoprotein metabolism. Fibrates have multiple effects on lipid and lipoprotein metabolism. All of these effects appear to be secondary to fibrates' action as agonists of the nuclear receptor, peroxisome proliferator-activated receptor α (PPAR α).[89] One of the major tissue locations of PPAR α is the liver, which is where fibrates have their major lipid effects.

As a result, the fibrates have multiple effects on serum lipoprotein levels. Among fibrates, fenofibrate has the most LDL-lowering potential. The greatest reductions in HDL cholesterol are seen in patients with elevated TG.[90]

Effects of fibrates, inflammation, and atherogenic pathways. Recent research suggests that activation of PPAR α by fibrates can occur in nonhepatic tissues (or cells). This has led to speculation that some of the potentially beneficial effects of fibrates could be through direct action on atherogenic processes.

Effects of fibrates on major coronary events. Several clinical trials have compared fibrates for coronary outcomes. Although reductions in CHD end points varied from trial to trial, there was a strong overall trend toward reduction in events. These findings are reinforced by angiographic trials, which collectively show less progression of coronary lesions in patients treated with fibrates.

Side effects of fibrates. The WHO clofibrate trial[91] suggests that clofibrate increases non-CHD mortality. This increase offsets any benefit from reduced CHD risk. Specific side effects were not identified in this trial. However, the findings impeded the use of fibrates for many years. Subsequent clinical trials have shown no increase in non-CHD mortality. Nonetheless, there are some side effects that must be recognized. These include GI distress, skin rashes, cholesterol gallstones, and myopathy. About 2% to 5% of patients treated with fibrates will develop cholesterol gallstones. Patients at risk for myopathy include those with end-stage renal disease and those taking statins. For the former, the dose of fibrates must be reduced according to the package insert for the drug. For concomitant use with statins, gemfibrozil should be avoided. The exceptionally high risk for myopathy with the combination of cerivastatin + gemfibrozil contributed to the removal of cerivastatin from the market.[92]

Whether used alone or combined with a statin, fibrates are not equivalent in their contribution to myopathy.[93,94] It appears that gemfibrozil interferes with statin catabolism, whereas fenofibrate does not.[95] Fenofibrate should therefore be less likely to induce myopathy in combination with statins than gemfibrozil. Fenofibrate also has the advantage of once-a-day dosing, and it is generally well tolerated.

Clinical use of fibrates in the metabolic syndrome. Fibrates are particularly useful in people with very high TG levels (>500 mg/dL) to reduce the risk for acute pancreatitis. Fenofibrate apparently has an advantage of safety over gemfibrozil when used in combination with statins in patients with atherogenic dyslipidemia.[72]

An important but unresolved issue is whether fibrates reduce risk for ASCVD events independent of their effects on plasma lipids. The favorable outcome of the VA-HIT trial particularly suggests such an effect, perhaps by mitigating the proinflammatory state. Furthermore, subgroup analysis of the VA-HIT trial suggests that the best results with gemfibrozil were obtained in people with characteristics of the metabolic syndrome (ie, hypertriglyceridemia, insulin resistance, and/or type 2 diabetes).[96,97] A similar result was obtained with gemfibrozil in the Helsinki Heart Study[98] and with bezafibrate in the Bezafibrate Infarction Prevention study.[99] If these results can be confirmed in studies with fenofibrate, the combination of statin and fenofibrate will be particularly attractive for patients with the metabolic syndrome.

Nicotinic Acid

Three forms of nicotinic acid are available: crystalline, sustained-release, and extended-release (Niaspan®).[71] Another preparation (Advicor®) combines extended-release niacin with lovastatin. Crystalline nicotinic acid is less expensive than the other types, but it must be taken 2 to 3 times per day and can cause unacceptable flushing. Sustained-release nicotinic acid generally does not cause flushing, but it is more likely to cause hepatotoxicity than the crystalline form. Niaspan® can be taken once a day and causes less flushing than crystalline nicotinic acid and less hepatotoxicity than sustained-release nicotinic acid. Crystalline and sustained-release nicotinic acid can be purchased over the counter or by prescription. Over-the-counter nicotinic acid is less expensive, but its purity cannot be assured. Niaspan® can be obtained only by prescription.

Effects on lipoprotein metabolism. Nicotinic acid, like fibrates, effectively lowers TG levels. Nicotinic acid also raises HDL-cholesterol levels[71] more than any other lipid-lowering drug. It also moderately lowers LDL levels. The mechanisms underlying these changes are not known. Nicotinic acid acutely suppresses release of nonesterified fatty acid (NEFA) from adipose tissue, but this change probably does not account for the drug's effect on lipoprotein metabolism. This effect is more likely secondary to metabolic changes in the liver.

Efficacy of nicotinic acid for reducing major coronary events. Limited clinical trial data indicate that nicotinic acid reduces the risk for major coronary events. The Coronary Drug Project (CDP)[100] was a secondary prevention trial in which nicotinic acid therapy reduced recurrence of CHD events by 25%. Long-term follow-up showed that patients who received nicotinic acid had a lower total mortality than did the placebo group. The Stockholm Ischemic Heart Disease Study[101] was another secondary prevention trial in which nicotinic acid was combined with clofibrate. In this trial, total CHD mortality was lowered by 36%. The greatest benefit was observed in the subgroup with higher TG levels. Several angiographic trials[71] revealed that combined drug therapy in which nicotinic acid was one of the agents reduced progression of coronary athero-sclerosis compared to control groups.

Side effects of nicotinic acid. Side effects include flushing, itching, skin rashes, GI distress, hepatotoxicity, hyperuricemia, and hyperglycemia. Thus, some patients who receive nicotinic acid cannot tolerate it on a long-term basis.

Use of nicotinic acid in patients with the metabolic syndrome. For efficacy of lipid lowering, nicotinic acid is an attractive agent to use in combination with statins in people with the metabolic syndrome. The combination mitigates all of the lipoprotein defects of atherogenic dyslipidemia: elevated levels of TGRLP, apo B, small LDL particles, and low HDL cholesterol. It is particularly efficacious for raising HDL levels. However, nicotinic acid can induce elevations of plasma glucose in some patients. Nicotinic acid can be used in patients with type 2 diabetes, but the dose should be kept low (1 to 2 g/d).[102]

When nicotinic acid is used in patients with the metabolic syndrome, several points of therapy should be remembered. If crystalline nicotinic acid is used, the initial dose should be very low (eg, 50 mg 3 times daily). The dose can then be doubled every 3 days up to about 1 g/d. The response in lipid and glucose levels should be rechecked. In a patient with the metabolic syndrome, the dose generally should not exceed 2 g/d. Long-acting nicotinic acid is not recommended because of increased risk for side effects.

References

1.   Genuth S, Alberti KG, Bennett P, et al: Follow-up report on the diagnosis of diabetes mellitus. The Expert Committee on the Diagnosis and Classification of Diabetes Mellitus. *Diabetes Care* 2003;26:3160-3167.

2.   Alberti KG, Zimmet PZ: Definition, diagnosis and classification of diabetes mellitus and its complications. Part 1: diagnosis and classification of diabetes mellitus: provisional report of a WHO consultation. *Diabet Med* 1998;15:539-553.

3.   American Diabetes Association. Standards of medical care in diabetes. *Diabetes Care* 2004;27(suppl 1):S15-S35.

4.   Grundy SM, Brewer HB Jr, Cleeman JI, et al: Definition of metabolic syndrome: report of the National Heart, Lung, and Blood Institute/American Heart Association conference on scientific issues related to definition. *Circulation* 2004;109:433-438.

5.   Knowler WC, Barrett-Connor E, Fowler SE, et al: Reduction in the incidence of type 2 diabetes with lifestyle intervention or metformin. *N Engl J Med* 2002;346:393-403.

6.   Wilhelmsen L, Pyorala K, Wedel H, et al: Risk factors for a major coronary event after myocardial infarction in the Scandinavian Simvastatin Survival Study (4S). Impact of predicted risk on the benefit of cholesterol-lowering treatment. *Eur Heart J* 2001; 22:1119-1127.

7.   Simes J, Furberg CD, Braunwald E, et al: Effects of pravastatin on mortality in patients with and without coronary heart disease across a broad range of cholesterol levels. The Prospective Pravastatin Pooling Project. *Eur Heart J* 2002;23:207-215.

8.   Migrino RQ, Topol EJ: A matter of life and death? The Heart Protection Study and protection of clinical trial participants. *Control Clin Trials* 2003;24:501-505.

9.   Robins SJ, Rubins HB, Faas FH, et al: Insulin resistance and cardiovascular events with low HDL cholesterol: the Veterans Affairs HDL Intervention Trial (VA-HIT). *Diabetes Care* 2003;26: 1513-1517.

10.   Effect of fenofibrate on progression of coronary-artery disease in type 2 diabetes: the Diabetes Atherosclerosis Intervention Study, a randomised study. *Lancet* 2001;357:905-910.

11.   Adler AI, Stratton IM, Neil HA, et al: Association of systolic blood pressure with macrovascular and microvascular complications of type 2 diabetes (UKPDS 36): prospective observational study. *BMJ* 2000;321:412-419.

12.   Droste DW, Ritter MA, Dittrich R, et al: Arterial hypertension and ischaemic stroke. *Acta Neurol Scand* 2003;107:241-251.

13.   Nesto RW, Bell D, Bonow RO, et al: Thiazolidinedione use, fluid retention, and congestive heart failure: a consensus statement from the American Heart Association and American Diabetes Association. October 7, 2003. *Circulation* 2003;108:2941-2948.

14. Lupi R, Del Guerra S, Fierabracci V, et al: Lipotoxicity in human pancreatic islets and the protective effect of metformin. *Diabetes* 2002;51(suppl 1):S134-S137.

15. Patane G, Piro S, Rabuazzo AM, et al: Metformin restores insulin secretion altered by chronic exposure to free fatty acids or high glucose: a direct metformin effect on pancreatic beta-cells. *Diabetes* 2000;49:735-740.

16. Ashcroft FM, Gribble FM: Tissue-specific effects of sulfonylureas: lessons from studies of cloned K(ATP) channels. *J Diabetes Complications* 2000;14:192-196.

17. Dunn CJ, Faulds D: Nateglinide. *Drugs* 2000;60:607-615.

18. Meinert CL, Knatterud GL, Prout TE, et al: A study of the effects of hypoglycemic agents on vascular complications in patients with adult-onset diabetes. II. Mortality results. *Diabetes* 1970;19(suppl):789-830.

19. Intensive blood-glucose control with sulphonylureas or insulin compared with conventional treatment and risk of complications in patients with type 2 diabetes (UKPDS 33). UK Prospective Diabetes Study (UKPDS) Group. *Lancet* 1998;352:837-853.

20. Riddle MC: Editorial: sulfonylureas differ in effects on ischemic preconditioning—is it time to retire glyburide? *J Clin Endocrinol Metab* 2003;88:528-530.

21. Skyler JS: Insulin therapy in type II diabetes: who needs it, how much of it, and for how long? *Postgrad Med* 1997;101:85-90, 92-94, 96.

22. The Seventh Report of the Joint National Committee on Prevention, Detection, Evaluation, and Treatment of High Blood Pressure. JNC VII. US Department of Health and Human Services National Institutes of Health National Heart, Lung, and Blood Institute, National High Blood Pressure Education Program. NIH Publication No. 03-5233. May, 2003.

23. Lewington S, Clarke R, Qizilbash N, et al: Age-specific relevance of usual blood pressure to vascular mortality: a meta-analysis of individual data for one million adults in 61 prospective studies. *Lancet* 2002;360:1903-1913.

24. Vasan RS, Beiser A, Seshadri S, et al: Residual lifetime risk for developing hypertension in middle-aged women and men: The Framingham Heart Study. *JAMA* 2002;287:1003-1010.

25. Neal B, MacMahon S, Chapman N: Effects of ACE inhibitors, calcium antagonists, and other blood-pressure-lowering drugs: Results of prospectively designed overviews of randomized trials. Blood Pressure Lowering Treatment Trialists' Collaboration. *Lancet* 2000;356:1955-1964.

26. Ogden LG, He J, Lydick E, et al: Long-term absolute benefit of lowering blood pressure in hypertensive patients according to the JNC VI risk stratification. *Hypertension* 2000;35: 539-543.

27. Birkenhäger WH, Staessen JA, Gasowski J, et al: Effects of antihypertensive treatment on endpoints in the diabetic patients randomized in the Systolic Hypertension in Europe (Syst-Eur) trial. *J Nephrol* 2000;13:232-237.

28. Zanchetti A, Hansson L, Clement D, et al: Benefits and risks of more intensive blood pressure lowering in hypertensive patients of the HOT study with different risk profiles: does a J-shaped curve exist in smokers? *J Hypertens* 2003;21:797-804.

29. Effects of ramipril on cardiovascular and microvascular outcomes in people with diabetes mellitus: results of the HOPE study and MICRO-HOPE substudy. Heart Outcomes Prevention Evaluation Study Investigators. *Lancet* 2000;355:253-259.

30. Lewis EJ, Hunsicker LG, Bain RP, et al: The effect of angiotensin-converting-enzyme inhibition on diabetic nephropathy. The Collaborative Study Group. *N Engl J Med* 1993;329:1456-1462.

31. Maschio G, Alberti D, Janin G, et al: Effect of the angiotensin-converting-enzyme inhibitor benazepril on the progression of chronic renal insufficiency. The Angiotensin-Converting-Enzyme Inhibition in Progressive Renal Insufficiency Study Group. *N Engl J Med* 1996;334:939-945.

32. Ravid M, Lang R, Rachmani R, et al: Long-term renoprotective effect of angiotensin-converting enzyme inhibition in non-insulin-dependent diabetes mellitus. A 7-year follow-up study. *Arch Intern Med* 1996;156:286-289.

33. Dahlof B, Devereux RB, Kjeldsen SE, et al: Cardiovascular morbidity and mortality in the Losartan Intervention For Endpoint reduction in hypertension study (LIFE): a randomised trial against atenolol. *Lancet* 2002;359:995-1003.

34. Lindholm LH, Ibsen H, Dahlof B, et al: Cardiovascular morbidity and mortality in patients with diabetes in the Losartan

Intervention For Endpoint reduction in hypertension study (LIFE): a randomised trial against atenolol. *Lancet* 2002;359:1004-1010.

35.   Tatti P, Pahor M, Byington RP, et al: Outcome results of the Fosinopril Versus Amlodipine Cardiovascular Events Randomized Trial (FACET) in patients with hypertension and NIDDM. *Diabetes Care* 1998;21:597-603.

36.   Hansson L, Lindholm LH, Niskanen L, et al: Effect of angiotensin-converting-enzyme inhibition compared with conventional therapy on cardiovascular morbidity and mortality in hypertension: the Captopril Prevention Project (CAPPP) randomised trial. *Lancet* 1999;353:611-616.

37.   Pahor M, Psaty BM, Alderman MH, et al: Therapeutic benefits of ACE inhibitors and other antihypertensive drugs in patients with type 2 diabetes. *Diabetes Care* 2000;23:888-892.

38.   O'Connor CM, Carson PE, Miller AB, et al: Effect of amlodipine on mode of death among patients with advanced heart failure in the PRAISE trial. Prospective Randomized Amlodipine Survival Evaluation. *Am J Cardiol* 1998;82:881-887.

39.   Sica DA, Douglas JG: The African American Study of Kidney Disease and Hypertension (AASK): new findings. *J Clin Hypertens* (Greenwich) 2001;3:244-251.

40.   Moser M: Why are physicians not prescribing diuretics more frequently in the management of hypertension? *JAMA* 1998; 279:1813-1816.

41.   Zanella MT, Kohlmann O Jr, Ribeiro AB: Treatment of obesity hypertension and diabetes syndrome. *Hypertension* 2001;38 (3 pt 2):705-708.

42.   Julius S, Majahalme S, Palatini P: Antihypertensive treatment of patients with diabetes and hypertension. *Am J Hypertens* 2001; 14(11 pt 2):310S-316S.

43.   Imazu M: Hypertension and insulin disorders. *Curr Hypertens Rep* 2002;4:477-482.

44.   Tourniaire J, Bajard L, Harfouch M, et al: [Restoration of insulin sensitivity after correction of hypokalemia due to chronic tubulopathy in a diabetic patient] *Diabete Metab* 1988;14:717-720. [Article in French]

45.   Wing LM, Reid CM, Ryan P, et al: A comparison of outcomes with angiotensin converting-enzyme inhibitors and diuretics for hypertension in the elderly. *N Engl J Med* 2003;348:583-592.

46. Psaty BM, Lumley T, Furberg CD, et al: Health outcomes associated with various antihypertensive therapies used as first-line agents: a network meta-analysis. *JAMA* 2003;289:2534-2544.

47. Soberman JE, Weber KT: Spironolactone in congestive heart failure. *Curr Hypertens Rep* 2000;2:451-456.

48. Pitt B, Williams G, Remme W, et al: The EPHESUS trial: eplerenone in patients with heart failure due to systolic dysfunction complicating acute myocardial infarction. Eplerenone Post-AMI Heart Failure Efficacy and Survival Study. *Cardiovasc Drugs Ther* 2001;15:79-87.

49. Brenner BM, Cooper ME, de Zeeuw D, et al: Effects of losartan on renal and cardiovascular outcomes in patients with type 2 diabetes and nephropathy. *N Engl J Med* 2001;345:861-869.

50. Lewis EJ, Hunsicker LG, Clarke WR, et al: Renoprotective effect of the angiotensin-receptor antagonist irbesartan in patients with nephropathy due to type 2 diabetes. *N Engl J Med* 2001;345: 851-860.

51. Gerth WC, Remuzzi G, Viberti G, et al: Losartan reduces the burden and cost of ESRD: public health implications from the RENAAL study for the European Union. *Kidney Int* 2002;62 (suppl 82):68-72.

52. Garg R, Yusuf S: Overview of randomized trials of angiotensin-converting enzyme inhibitors on mortality and morbidity in patients with heart failure. Collaborative Group on ACE Inhibitor Trials. *JAMA* 1995;273:1450-1456.

53. Cohn JN, Tognoni G, Valsartan Heart Failure Trial Investigators: A randomized trial of the angiotensin-receptor blocker valsartan in chronic heart failure. *N Engl J Med* 2001;345:1667-1675.

54. Struckman DR, Rivey MP: Combined therapy with an angiotensin II receptor blocker and an angiotensin-converting enzyme inhibitor in heart failure. *Ann Pharmacother* 2001;35:242-248.

55. Cohn JN: Interaction of beta-blockers and angiotensin receptor blockers/ACE inhibitors in heart failure. *J Renin Angiotensin Aldosterone Syst* 2003;4:137-139.

56. Dimopoulos K, Salukhe TV, Coats AJ, et al: Meta-analyses of mortality and morbidity effects of an angiotensin receptor blocker in patients with chronic heart failure already receiving an ACE inhibitor (alone or with a beta-blocker). *Int J Cardiol* 2004;93: 105-111.

57. Padwal R, Laupacis A: Antihypertensive therapy and incidence of type 2 diabetes: a systematic review. *Diabetes Care* 2004; 27:247-255.

58. Brook RD: Mechanism of differential effects of antihypertensive agents on serum lipids. *Curr Hypertens Rep* 2000;2: 370-377.

59. ALLHAT Collaborative Research Group: Major cardiovascular events in hypertensive patients randomized to doxazosin vs chlorthalidone: the antihypertensive and lipid-lowering treatment to prevent heart attack trial (ALLHAT). *JAMA* 2000;283:1967-1975.

60. Landsberg L, Young JB: Physiology and pharmacology of the autonomic nervous system. In: *Harrison's Principles of Internal Medicine*, 14th ed. Isselbacher K et al, eds. New York, McGraw-Hill, 1998.

61. Foster DW, Rubenstein AH: Hypoglycemia. In: *Harrison's Principles of Internal Medicine*, 14th ed. Isselbacher K et al, eds. New York, McGraw-Hill, 1998.

62. Tight blood pressure control and risk of macrovascular and microvascular complications in type 2 diabetes: UKPDS 38. UK Prospective Diabetes Study Group. *BMJ* 1998;317:703-713.

63. Bakris GL, Fonseca V, Katholi RE, et al: Metabolic effects of carvedilol vs metoprolol in patients with type 2 diabetes mellitus and hypertension: a randomized controlled trial. *JAMA* 2004;292: 2227-2236.

64. Sowers JR: SUNY School of Medicine. Personal communication.

65. The ALLHAT Officers and Coordinators for the ALLHAT Collaborative Research Group: The Antihypertensive and Lipid-Lowering Treatment to Prevent Heart Attack Trial (ALLHAT). Major outcomes in high-risk hypertensive patients randomized to angiotensin converting enzyme inhibitor or calcium channel blocker vs diuretic: The Antihypertensive and Lipid-Lowering Treatment to Prevent Heart Attack Trial (ALLHAT). *JAMA* 2002; 288:2981-2997.

66. Williams GH: Hypertensive vascular disease. In: *Harrison's Principles of Internal Medicine*, 14th ed. Isselbacher K et al, eds. New York, McGraw-Hill, 1998.

67. Drug Facts and Comparisons. St Louis, 2000.

68. Jukema JW, van der Hoorn JW: Amlodipine and atorvastatin in atherosclerosis: a review of the potential of combination therapy. *Expert Opin Pharmacother* 2004;5:459-468.

69. Jukema JW, Zwinderman AH, van Boven AJ, et al: Evidence for a synergistic effect of calcium channel blockers with lipid-lowering therapy in retarding progression of coronary atherosclerosis in symptomatic patients with normal to moderately raised cholesterol levels. The REGRESS Study Group. *Arterioscler Thromb Vasc Biol* 1996;16:425-430.

70. Liebovitz E, Beniashvili M, Zimlichmn R, et al: Treatment with amlodipine and atorvastatin has additive effect in improvement of arterial compliance in hypertensive hyperlipidemic patients. *Am J Hypertens* 2003;(9 pt 1):715-718.

71. Third Report of the National Cholesterol Education Program (NCEP) Expert Panel on Detection, Evaluation, and Treatment of High Blood Cholesterol in Adults (Adult Treatment Panel III) final report. *Circulation* 2002;106:3143-3421.

72. Vega GL, Ma PT, Cater NB, et al: Effects of adding feno-fibrate (200 mg/day) to simvastatin (10 mg/day) in patients with combined hyperlipidemia and metabolic syndrome. *Am J Cardiol* 2003;91:956-960.

73. Ballantyne CM, Olsson AG, Cook TJ, et al: Influence of low high-density lipoprotein cholesterol and elevated triglyceride on coronary heart disease events and response to simvastatin therapy in 4S. *Circulation* 2001;104:3046-3051.

74. Grundy SM: HMG-CoA reductase inhibitors for treatment of hypercholesterolemia. *N Engl J Med* 1988;319:24-33.

75. Endo A: The discovery and development of HMG CoA reductase inhibitors. *J Lipid Res* 1992;33:1569-1582.

76. Shepherd J, Cobbe SM, Ford I, et al: Prevention of coronary heart disease with pravastatin in men with hypercholesterolemia.West of Scotland Coronary Prevention Study Group. *N Engl J Med* 1995;333:1301-1307.

77. Downs JR, Clearfield M, Weis S, et al: Primary prevention of acute coronary events with lovastatin in men and women with average cholesterol levels: results of AFCAPS/TexCAPS. Air Force/Texas Coronary Atherosclerosis Prevention Study. *JAMA* 1998;279:1615-1622.

78.   Sever PS, Dahlof B, Poulter NR, et al: Prevention of coronary and stroke events with atorvastatin in hypertensive patients who have average or lower-than-average cholesterol concentrations, in the Anglo-Scandinavian Cardiac Outcomes Trial—Lipid Lowering Arm (ASCOT-LLA): a multicentre randomised controlled trial. *Lancet* 2003;361:1149-1158.

79.   Heart Protection Study Collaborative Group: MRC/BHF Heart Protection Study of cholesterol lowering with simvastatin in 20,536 high-risk individuals: a randomised placebo-controlled trial. *Lancet* 2002;360:7-22.

80.   Shepherd J, Blauw GJ, Murphy MB, et al: Pravastatin in elderly individuals at risk of vascular disease (PROSPER): a randomised controlled trial. *Lancet* 2002;360:1623-1630.

81.   Pasternak RC, Smith SC Jr, Bairey-Merz CN, et al: ACC/AHA/NHLBI Clinical Advisory on the use and safety of statins. *Circulation* 2002;106:1024-1028.

82.   Miettinen TA, Puska P, Gylling H, et al: Reduction of serum cholesterol with sitostanol-ester margarine in a mildly hypercholesterolemic population. *N Engl J Med* 1995;333:1308-1312.

83.   Plat J, van Onselen EN, van Heugten MM, et al: Effects on serum lipids, lipoproteins and fat soluble antioxidant concentrations of consumption frequency of margarines and shortenings enriched with plant stanol esters. *Eur J Clin Nutr* 2000;54: 671-677.

84.   Ballantyne CM, Houri J, Notarbartolo A, et al: Effect of ezetimibe coadministered with atorvastatin in 628 patients with primary hypercholesterolemia: a prospective, randomized, double-blind trial. *Circulation* 2003;107:2409-2415.

85.   Grundy SM: Alternative approaches to cholesterol-lowering therapy. *Am J Cardiol* 2002;90:1135-1138.

86.   The Lipid Research Clinics Coronary Primary Prevention Trial Results: I. Reduction in the incidence of coronary heart disease. *JAMA* 1984;251:351-364.

87.   Bays H, Dujovne C: Colesevelam HCl: a non-systemic lipid-altering drug. *Expert Opin Pharmacother* 2003;4:779-790.

88.   Garg A, Grundy SM: Cholestyramine therapy for dyslipidemia in non-insulin-dependent diabetes mellitus. A short-term, double-blind, crossover trial. *Ann Intern Med* 1994;121:416-422.

89. Lee CH, Olson P, Evans RM: Minireview: lipid metabolism, metabolic diseases, and peroxisome proliferator-activated receptors. *Endocrinology* 2003;144:2201-2207.

90. Steinmetz A, Schwartz T, Hehnke U, et al: Multicenter comparison of micronized fenofibrate and simvastatin in patients with primary type IIA or IIb hyperlipoproteinemia. *J Cardiovasc Pharmacol* 1996;27:563-570.

91. A co-operative trial in the primary prevention of ischemic heart disease using clofibrate. Report from the Committee of Principal Investigators. *Br Heart J* 1978;40:1069-1118.

92. Staffa JA, Chang J, Green L: Cerivastatin and reports of fatal rhabdomyolysis. *N Engl J Med* 2002;346:539-540.

93. Duell PB, Connor WE, Illingworth DR: Rhabdomyolysis after taking atorvastatin with gemfibrozil. *Am J Cardiol* 1998;81:368-369.

94. Wierzbicki AS, Lumb PJ, Cheung J, et al: Fenofibrate plus simvastatin therapy versus simvastatin plus cholestyramine therapy for familial hypercholesterolemia. *QJM* 1997;90:631-634.

95. Pan WJ, Gustavson LE, Achari R, et al: Lack of a clinically significant pharmacokinetic interaction between fenofibrate and pravastatin in healthy volunteers. *J Clin Pharmacol* 2000;40:316-323.

96. Rubins HB, Robins SJ, Collins D, et al: Diabetes, plasma insulin, and cardiovascular disease: subgroup analysis from the Department of Veterans Affairs high-density lipoprotein intervention trial (VA-HIT). *Arch Intern Med* 2002;162:2597-2604.

97. Robins SJ, Rubins HB, Faas FH, et al: Insulin resistance and cardiovascular events with low HDL cholesterol: the Veterans Affairs HDL Intervention Trial (VA-HIT). *Diabetes Care* 2003;26:1513-1517.

98. Tenkanen L, Manttari M, Manninen V: Some coronary risk factors related to the insulin resistance syndrome and treatment with gemfibrozil. Experience from the Helsinki Heart Study. *Circulation* 1995;92:1779-1785.

99. Secondary prevention by raising HDL cholesterol and reducing triglycerides in patients with coronary artery disease: the Bezafibrate Infarction Prevention (BIP) Study. *Circulation* 2000;102:21-27.

100. Clofibrate and niacin in coronary heart disease. *JAMA* 1975;231:360-381.

101. Carlson LA, Rosenhamer G: Reduction of mortality in the Stockholm Ischaemic Heart Disease Secondary Prevention Study by combined treatment with clofibrate and nicotinic acid. *Acta Med Scand* 1988;223:405-418.

102. Grundy SM, Vega GL, McGovern ME, et al: Efficacy, safety, and tolerability of once-daily niacin for the treatment of dyslipidemia associated with type 2 diabetes: results of the assessment of diabetes control and evaluation of the efficacy of niaspan trial. *Arch Intern Med* 2002;162:1568-1576.

Chapter **5**

Classification and Pathogenesis of the Post-MI Patient

Despite major advances in the treatment and prevention of coronary heart disease (CHD) that have reduced its incidence during the past 4 decades, CHD caused by coronary atherosclerosis continues to surpass all other causes of mortality in industrialized societies. The grim toll of CHD in the United States is reflected by more than 500,000 deaths each year and by a cost of more than $20 billion in medical care for the 14 million patients with one or more forms of the disease.[1] The annual incidence of acute myocardial infarction (AMI) in the United States is estimated at 1.2 million to 1.5 million cases, of which more than one third are fatal before the victim reaches a hospital. However, of those who are hospitalized, survival has steadily risen from 70% 30 years ago to approximately 90% today. Thus, almost 1 million patients stricken with AMI survive and are discharged from the hospital annually. This group, which is at high risk for recurrent events, has benefited from recent therapeutic innovations, including cardioprotective drugs, myocardial revascularization, cardiac services, and lifestyle changes. These innovations have significantly improved long-term prognosis after AMI.

Optimal management of the post-MI patient requires (1) a systematic approach to assess the risk for recurrent coronary events; and (2) appropriate application of the growing number of therapeutic options that have had a favorable effect on prognosis. The foundation of this strategy is an understanding of current concepts of the pathophysiology of CHD and its complications.

The Spectrum of Coronary Heart Disease

Coronary artery disease produces a number of clinical syndromes that comprise the spectrum of CHD, of which AMI is the most frequent initial manifestation. The other major clinical presentations of CHD are angina pectoris and sudden death. Estimates vary, but current data suggest that AMI is the initial expression of CHD in 40% to 50% of patients. Angina pectoris is the first indication of the disease in 30% to 40% of patients; sudden death (defined as death within 1 hour of onset of symptoms) is the presenting finding in 10% to 20% of CHD victims.

Additional complications of CHD include unstable angina (UA) (which is occasionally CHD's first manifestation), arrhythmias, and congestive heart failure (CHF). The latter is usually related to extensive loss of myocardium from one or more MIs. A striking message of these statistics is that the initial presentation of CHD in most patients is a human catastrophe: MI or sudden death. Furthermore, angina pectoris is the first clinical finding in a minority of patients. Thus, primary prevention on a wide scale is obviously needed to achieve a major reduction in the burden of CHD.

Traditional Classification

The most common symptom of myocardial ischemia is chest discomfort. When this symptom is severe and prolonged (ie, >20 minutes), AMI or UA should be considered. The diagnosis of MI continues to be based on at least two of the following three major clinical findings: compatible symptoms (usually typical chest discomfort), electrocardiographic evidence of ischemia/injury, and/or

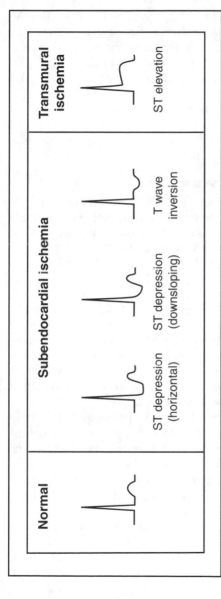

Figure 5-1: Common transient electrocardiogram abnormalities during ischemia. Subendocardial ischemia results in ST-segment depressions and/or T-wave flattening or inversions. Severe transient transmural ischemia can result in ST-segment elevations, similar to the early changes in AMI. When transient ischemia resolves, so do the electrocardiographic changes. Reproduced with permission from Sabatine MS, O'Gara PT, Lilly LS: Ischemic heart disease. In: Lilly LS, ed. *Pathophysiology of Heart Disease*, 2nd ed. Baltimore, MD, Lippincott Williams & Wilkins, 1998, p 134.[2]

evolution of pathologic Q waves, and characteristic changes in serum markers of cardiac injury.[3] MI was traditionally categorized as transmural or nontransmural (or subendocardial), based on the presence or absence, respectively, of pathologic Q waves on the electrocardiogram (ECG). In the absence of ECG evolution of pathologic Q waves (40 msec duration), elevations of serum markers of cardiac injury were required for the diagnosis of nontransmural MI, while UA was indicated if there was no elevation of serum markers.

Contemporary Classification

Although it does not differ fundamentally from the traditional categories, the current classification of the acute ischemic manifestations of CHD is based on improved understanding of the underlying pathophysiology. Acute myocardial ischemia/infarction is now viewed as a continuum from UA to non-Q-wave MI (NQMI) and Q-wave MI (QwMI). These disorders are collectively considered the acute coronary syndromes (ACS).[4] Clinicians recognize the limitations of former classifications relating the ECG to MI pathology in that Q-wave MI is not consistently transmural nor is non-Q-wave MI always nontransmural. Moreover, the development of increasingly sensitive serum markers of cardiac injury, such as the troponins, has blurred the distinction between NQMI and UA.

All ACS are characterized by prolonged chest pain compatible with myocardial ischemia/infarction. The diagnosis of each is based on subsequent ECG alterations and serum marker data.[4] Q-wave MI is recognized in its early stages by ST-segment elevation (STE) and is, therefore, termed STEMI (Figure 5-1).[2] Non-Q-wave MI is referred to as non-STEMI, or NSTEMI ACS. Both STEMI and NSTEMI are, by definition, associated with elevation of serum markers of myocardial injury. In NSTEMI ACS, the ECG may show ST depression, T-wave inversion, or it may be normal (Figure 5-2). Absence of the latter in

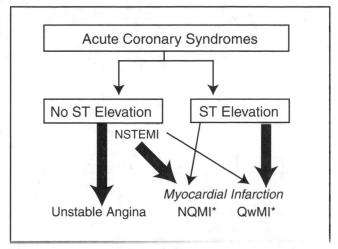

Figure 5-2: Nomenclature of acute coronary syndromes (ACS). Patients with ischemic discomfort may present with or without ST-segment elevation (STE) on the ECG. Most patients with STE (large arrows) ultimately develop a Q-wave acute myocardial infarction (QwMI), whereas a minority (small arrows) develop a non-Q-wave AMI (NQMI). Patients who present without STE are experiencing either UA or a non-ST-elevation MI (NSTEMI). The distinction between these two diagnoses is ultimately made based on the presence or absence of a cardiac marker detected in the blood.

*Elevation of cardiac injury marker.

Reproduced with permission from Antman EM, Braunwald E: Acute myocardial infarction. In: Braunwald E, ed. *Heart Disease: A Textbook of Cardiovascular Medicine*, 5th ed, vol 2. Philadelphia, PA, WB Saunders, 1997, pp 1184-1288.[5]

NSTEMI defines UA. These relationships are depicted in Figure 5-2. Refined diagnostic methods for detecting cardiac injury have confirmed the continuous nature of myo-

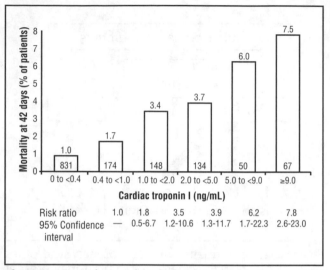

Figure 5-3: Relationship between cardiac troponin I levels and risk of mortality in patients with acute coronary syndromes. Reproduced with permission from Antman et al, *N Engl J Med* 1996;335:1342-1349.[6]

cardial ischemia/infarction, resulting in the concept of minimal myocardial damage for borderline elevations of the troponins, currently the most sensitive and specific indicators of myocardial injury. The arbitrary classification of UA and NQMI, which are part of the continuum of CHD, is also reflected by the direct correlation of mortality with the degree of elevation of the troponins in NSTEMI. This is indicated in Figure 5-3,[6] which demonstrates that mortality begins to rise with even small elevations of the troponins.

Pathogenesis of Acute Myocardial Infarction
Plaque Rupture

Myocardial infarction is the irreversible necrosis of cardiac muscle that results from an inadequate oxygen supply caused by the interruption of coronary blood flow to the myocardium. Infarction can involve any chamber of the heart, but it most frequently occurs in the left ventricle because of its high oxygen requirements, which considerably surpass those of the other cardiac chambers. In approximately 90% of patients with AMI, this impairment of blood supply is the result of acute thrombotic obstruction of a coronary artery. Recent studies indicate that coronary thrombosis is initiated by rupture of an atherosclerotic plaque that induces a cascade of vasculo-occlusive mechanisms.[7] Plaque rupture exposes the thrombogenic subendothelial collagen matrix, which induces local aggregation of platelets, promoting superimposition of fibrin deposition to form a thrombus at the site of ulceration. Activated platelets release factors, such as thromboxane A_2 and serotonin, that provoke vasospasm and augment platelet activity, inducing further aggregation, hemostasis, and thrombogenesis. These pathogenic mechanisms overwhelm endogenous vasodilator and antithrombotic factors, such as prostacyclin and tissue plasminogen activator, whose production by diseased endothelium is inadequate to offset the intense thrombotic activity initiated by plaque rupture.

Evolution and Extent of Myocardial Infarction

Coronary thrombosis is usually acute but may evolve over minutes or many hours, depending on the degree of imbalance between prothrombotic and antithrombotic mechanisms at the site of plaque rupture. However, for myocardial necrosis to occur, the imbalance between myocardial oxygen requirements and oxygen supply must be severe and prolonged. Infarction is a dynamic process, with myocardial necrosis usually progressing to completion in a jeopardized region over 6 to 8 hours after interruption of blood supply (Figure 5-4).[5] The interval varies, depending on the determinants of myocardial oxygen demand (heart rate, blood pressure, contractility, ventricu-

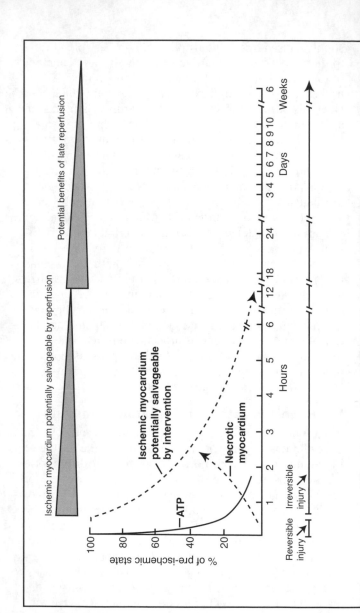

Figure 5-4: Temporal sequence of early biochemical, ultrastructural, histochemical, and histologic findings after onset of myocardial infarction. At the top of the figure, schematically shown, are the time frames for early and late reperfusion of the myocardium supplied by an occluded coronary artery. For approximately one half hour following the onset of even the most severe ischemia, myocardial injury is potentially reversible; after that, there is progressive loss of viability that is complete by 6 to 12 hours. The benefits of reperfusion (early and late) are greatest when it is achieved early, with progressively smaller benefits occurring as reperfusion is delayed. Reproduced with permission from Gersh BJ, Braunwald E, Bonow RO: Chronic coronary artery disease. In: Braunwald E, ed. *Heart Disease: A Textbook of Cardiovascular Medicine*, 5th ed, vol 2. Philadelphia, PA, WB Saunders, 1997, pp 1184-1288.[5]

			TTC staining defect →			
Electron microscopy	Glycogen depletion; mitochondrial swelling; relaxation of myofibrils	Sarcolemmal disruption: mitochondrial amorphous densities				
Histochemistry						
Light microscopy		Waviness of fibers at border	Beginning coagulation necrosis; edema; focal hemorrhage; beginning neutrophilic infiltrate	Continuing coagulation necrosis; pallor (shrunken nuclei and eosinophilic cytoplasm); myocsite contraction bands	Coagulation necrosis with loss of nuclei and striations; neutrophilic infiltrate	Disintegration of myofibers and phagocytosis by macrophages	Completion of phagocytosis; prominent granulation tissue with neovascularization and fibrovascular reaction
Gross changes				Pallor	Pallor, sometimes hyperemia; yellowing at periphery	Hyperemic border, central yellow-brown softening	Maximally yellow and soft vascularized edges; red-brown and depressed	Mature fibrous scar

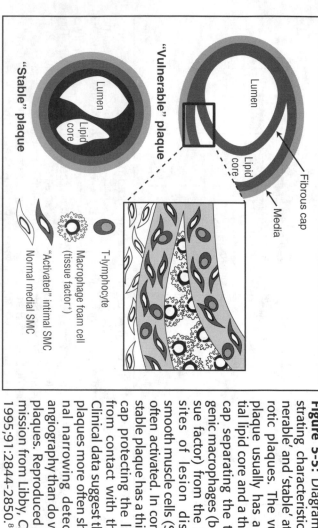

Figure 5-5: Diagram demonstrating characteristics of 'vulnerable' and 'stable' atherosclerotic plaques. The vulnerable plaque usually has a substantial lipid core and a thin fibrous cap separating the thrombogenic macrophages (bearing tissue factor) from the blood. At sites of lesion disruption, smooth muscle cells (SMCs) are often activated. In contrast, the stable plaque has a thick fibrous cap protecting the lipid core from contact with the blood. Clinical data suggest that stable plaques more often show luminal narrowing detectable by angiography than do vulnerable plaques. Reproduced with permission from Libby, *Circulation* 1995;91:2844-2850.[8]

122

lar volume) and oxygen supply (collateral coronary arteries, arterial pO_2, diastolic time interval, diastolic coronary perfusion gradient) during the coronary occlusive process. An understanding of these factors provides the basis for contemporary management of AMI, the primary goal of which is limiting the extent of myocardial injury and thereby reducing MI size. The importance of this objective is reflected by the fact that MI size, or the amount of myocardial damage, is one of the primary determinants, if not *the* primary determinant, of short-term and long-term clinical outcome.[10]

Vulnerable and Stable Plaques

Knowledge of the pathophysiology of AMI indicates why this drastic clinical event is so often the initial manifestation of CHD without prior warning by a less severe clinical syndrome such as stable angina. According to current concepts, the plaque that ulcerates and sets in motion the cascade of thrombogenesis and coronary occlusion possesses a thin fibrous cap and a large lipid pool (Figure 5-5).[7,9] It is also the site of multiple mediators of inflammation that promote ulceration and rupture of the fibrous cap. Because it is prone to rupture, it is referred to as a vulnerable plaque. In contrast, a stable plaque is characterized by a thick fibrous cap and a relatively small lipid pool, has little evidence of inflammatory activity, and is less subject to ulceration with consequent coronary thrombosis. The vulnerable plaque is typically noncritical in terms of the degree of coronary stenosis it produces in its quiescent state, which is usually less than 70% reduction of lumen diameter. Symptoms of myocardial ischemia do not usually occur with this degree of stenosis because it does not significantly impair coronary blood flow at rest or augmentation with stress. Reduction of the latter (coronary blood flow reserve) is associated with stenoses 70% or more, while impairment of resting coronary flow occurs when lumen diameter is reduced by >90%. These

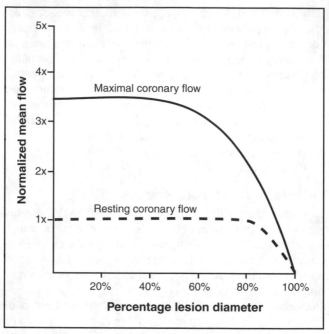

Figure 5-6: Resting and maximal coronary blood flow are affected by the magnitude of proximal arterial stenosis (percentage lesion diameter). The dotted line indicates resting blood flow, and the solid line represents maximal blood flow (ie, when there is a full dilatation of the distal resistance vessels). Compromise of maximal blood flow is evident when the proximal stenosis reduces the coronary lumen diameter by more than ~70%. Resting flow may be compromised if the stenosis exceeds ~90%. Reproduced with permission from Gould et al, *Am J Cardiol* 1974;34:48-55.[10]

relationships are depicted in Figure 5-6.[10] Most vulnerable plaques are clinically 'silent' until rupture and thrombosis occur. These findings further emphasize the importance of prevention of atherosclerosis in combating CHD.

Pathophysiology of the Acute Coronary Syndromes

The degree of thrombotic coronary obstruction typically determines which form of ACS ensues after plaque ulceration and coronary thrombosis.[7] A totally occlusive thrombus completely interrupts regional myocardial blood flow, resulting in STEMI and, usually, substantial myocardial necrosis. A partially occlusive thrombus produces incomplete reduction of coronary blood flow and severe myocardial ischemia, resulting in either NSTEMI (elevation of serum markers) or UA (no elevation of serum markers). The degree of elevation of serum markers in ACS generally, but not always, correlates with the extent of myocardial damage and, therefore, with morbidity and mortality (Figure 5-3).[6]

As previously stated, there is a general correlation between the pathogenesis of MI and the extent of myocardial damage. Because NSTEMI usually involves less cardiac muscle loss than STEMI, mortality and other serious complications, such as cardiogenic shock, CHF, and serious arrhythmias, are less common during the initial hospitalization in the former than the latter. However, in some cases, NSTEMI may result in extensive damage and STEMI may be associated with lesser injury. Furthermore, recurrent events are common with NSTEMI. In this regard, it has been shown that early mortality in STEMI and NSTEMI ACS varies much less than long-term mortality, which is actually higher after NSTEMI (Figure 5-7).[11] This finding has been attributed to factors such as greater extent of CAD, prior MI, and less intensive therapy of NSTEMI patients. Infarct size is also related to additional factors, such as the specific 'culprit' coronary artery, the site of vessel occlusion, presence of collateral coronary arteries, and the hemodynamic factors influencing myocardial oxygen demand and supply during the evolution of the infarction.

Nonatherosclerotic Causes of Myocardial Infarction

Although uncommon, MI can occur in the absence of coronary atherosclerosis. Nonatherosclerotic etiologies in-

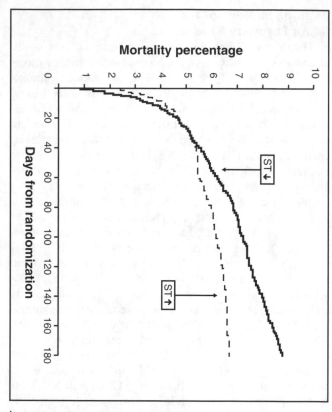

Figure 5-7: Kaplan-Meier estimates of 6-month mortality in patients with ST-elevation MI and those with acute coronary syndrome associated with ST depression. Adapted with permission from Savonitto S, Ardissino D, Granger CB, et al: Prognostic value of the admission electrocardiogram in acute coronary syndromes. *JAMA* 1999;281:707-713.[11]

clude coronary vasospasm, coronary emboli, vasculitis, congenital anomalies, trauma, and excessive myocardial oxygen demand in the presence of normal coronary arteries. The latter derangement can occur with cocaine abuse (vasospasm as well as hypertension and tachycardia), severe aortic stenosis, and hypertrophic obstructive cardiomyopathy. Cocaine and other drugs of abuse, such as methamphetamines, should be considered in young patients presenting with ACS, particularly those with few or no cardiovascular risk factors. These agents can be screened for by urine toxicology studies on admission.

Diagnosis of Acute Myocardial Infarction

Diagnosis of ACS among the 8 million patients presenting to emergency departments with chest pain each year in the United States is a continuing challenge. In most patients, this symptom is not related to acute cardiovascular disease and they are increasingly managed in chest pain units for low-risk patients. These patients are recognized by normal ECGs and negative cardiac injury markers.[12]

Recent guidelines of the American College of Cardiology and the American Heart Association (ACC/AHA) provide recommendations for management of ACS according to current standards of care, based on clinical evidence of efficacy. As stated earlier, diagnosis of AMI continues to be based on at least two of the following factors:

(1) Compatible symptoms, which usually consist of pressure-like retrosternal discomfort. Other presentations, such as dyspnea and mental status changes, are not uncommon, particularly in women and the elderly.

(2) ECG alterations of injury consisting of ST-segment elevation (Figure 5-1),[2] which may or may not evolve with the development of pathologic Q waves. This depends on the timeliness of therapy, particularly coronary reperfusion. Other ECG changes, such as ST-segment depression and T-wave inversion, are consistent with is-

chemia but have many other possible causes. They can provide further evidence of ACS in patients with compatible clinical presentations.

(3) Evolution of serum markers of cardiac injury, which is now based primarily on troponin I or T because of their superior sensitivity and specificity for detecting infarction. Because of the prolonged elevation of the troponins (7 to 14 days) after MI, measurement of the MB fraction of creatine kinase remains useful for identifying early reinfarction.

Management of Acute Myocardial Infarction

The initial management of AMI entails a comprehensive approach with the goals of early relief of symptoms and prevention of mortality and morbidity related to the acute event.[3] In survivors of MI, the objectives are long-term prevention of recurrent events and restoration of optimal functional status. Modern management of AMI is based on rapid diagnosis and early institution of therapy. Current recommendations include obtaining and interpreting an ECG within 10 minutes in all adults presenting to the emergency department with symptoms consistent with ACS, most typically chest discomfort.

ST-elevation Myocardial Infarction

For patients with ST-segment elevation and no contraindications, pharmacologic reperfusion therapy should be initiated within 30 minutes of presentation. If a short-acting thrombolytic agent is used, heparin should be administered as adjunctive therapy. Recent evidence indicates that clopidogrel (Plavix®) added to thrombolytic therapy significantly reduces mortality in STEMI.[13,14] Additionally, in patients with LVEF cardiac events posthospitalization, less than 40% are reduced by carvedilol (Coreg®).[15] Other medications administered at initial presentation include oxygen and aspirin. Analgesia should be used if indicated. In the absence of contraindications, patients should receive a nitrate and a β-blocker. An ACE inhibitor should be added early (first or second day). Use of this battery of medications assumes no contraindications to these agents, which may include low blood pressure (nitrates, β-blocker, ACE inhibitor) or low heart rate (β-blocker). Based on recent data, one of the statins can also be administered early in the course of infarction to initiate the benefits of lipid lowering early and to capitalize on statins' potential anti-inflammatory actions during the acute phase of MI. In hospitals with cardiac catheterization laboratories and expertise in acute coronary intervention, the preferred method for coronary reperfusion is primary angioplasty with stent placement. Coronary stent placement also involves short-term administration of a platelet glycoprotein IIB/IIIA inhibitor for optimal stent patency. Reduction of mortality and morbidity of 20% to 35% in patients with AMI has been demonstrated with the use of reperfusion therapy (pharmacologic or angioplasty), aspirin, β-blockers, and ACE inhibitors.

Non-ST-elevation Acute Coronary Syndromes

If the patient presenting with chest pain has NSTEMI ACS, based on cardiac serum markers and/or ECG changes, initial therapy includes aspirin, heparin, nitrates, and a β-blocker. Recent findings indicate that clopidogrel reduces combined ischemic events in NSTEMI ACS and, therefore, should be added to initial treatment.[16] An ACE inhibitor and a statin are also important components of early therapy. If this management fails to alleviate symptoms and/or ischemia, more intensive therapy involves addition of a platelet IIB/IIIA inhibitor and/or coronary intervention. It should be stated that in most patients with NSTEMI ACS, intensive medical therapy provides appropriate initial management. Although most clinical trials have favored the invasive approach for reducing future major adverse cardiac events, the most recent of these (ICTUS) reported comparable clinical outcomes with both strategies.[17]

Post-acute Hospital Phase

Overall survival in patients reaching the hospital with AMI is approximately 90%. However, this varies widely and may be close to 100% in the lowest-risk patients (young patients with small, uncomplicated MIs) and <50% in the highest-risk group (elderly patients with large, complicated MIs). Posthospital management entails secondary prevention by risk factor reduction, use of cardioprotective drugs (eg, aspirin, clopidogrel, β-blockers, ACE inhibitors, statins). Patients who are at high risk based on continuing symptoms or evidence of residual major cardiac ischemia on noninvasive testing should undergo cardiac catheterization and, if indicated, myocardial revascularization.[3,4]

References

1. American Heart Association: Heart Disease and Stroke Statistics—2004 update. Dallas, TX.

2. Sabatine MS, O'Gara PT, Lilly PS: Ischemic heart disease. In: Lilly LS, ed: *Pathophysiology of Heart Disease*, 2nd ed. Baltimore, MD, Lippincott Williams & Wilkins, 1998, p 134.

3. Antman EM, Anbe DT, Armstrong PW, et al: ACC/AHA guidelines for the management of patients with ST-elevation myocardial infarction: a report of the American College of Cardiology/ American Heart Association Task Force on Practice Guidelines (Committee to Revise the 1999 Guidelines for the Management of Patients with Acute Myocardial Infarction). *Circulation* 2004; 110:e82-e292.

4. Braunwald E, Antman EM, Beasley JW, et al: ACC/AHA 2002 guideline update for the management of patients with unstable angina and non-ST-segment elevation myocardial infarction—summary article: a report of the American College of Cardiology/American Heart Association task force on practice guidelines (Committee on the Management of Patients With Unstable Angina). *J Am Coll Cardiol* 2002;40:1366-1374.

5. Antman EM, Braunwald EM: Acute myocardial infarction. In: Braunwald E, ed. *Heart Disease: A Textbook of Cardiovascular Medicine*, 5th ed, vol 2. Philadelphia, PA, WB Saunders Co, 1997, pp 1184-1288.

6. Antman EM, Tanasijevic MJ, Thompson B, et al: Cardiac-specific troponin I levels to predict the risk of mortality in patients with acute coronary syndromes. *N Engl J Med* 1996;335:1342-1349.

7. Libby, P: Current concepts of the pathogenesis of the acute coronary syndromes. *Circulation* 2001;104:365-372.

8. Libby P: Molecular bases of the acute coronary syndromes. *Circulation* 1995;91:2844-2850.

9. Phibbs B, Marcus F, Marriott HJ, et al: Q-wave versus non-Q-wave myocardial infarction: a meaningless distinction. *J Am Coll Cardiol* 1999;335:576-582.

10. Gould KL, Lipscomb K: Effects of coronary stenoses on coronary flow reserve and resistance. *Am J Cardiol* 1974;34:48-55.

11. Savonitto S, Ardissino D, Granger CB, et al: Prognostic value of the admission electrocardiogram in acute coronary syndromes. *JAMA* 1999;281:707-713.

12. Diercks DB, Kirk JD, Amersterdam EA: Chest pain units: management of special populations. *Cardiol Clin* 2005;23:549-557.

13. Sabatine MS, Cannon CP, Gibson CM, et al: Addition of clopidogrel to aspirin and fibrinolytic therapy for myocardial infarction with ST-segment elevation. *N Engl J Med* 2005;352:1179-1189.

14. Chen ZM, Pan HC, Chen YP, et al: Early intravenous then oral metoprolol in 45,852 patients with acute myocardial infarction: a randomised placebo-controlled trial. COMMIT (Clopidogrel and Metoprolol in Myocardial Infarction Trial) collaborative group. *Lancet* 2005;366:1622-1632.

15. Dargie HJ: Effect of carvedilol on outcome after myocardial infarction in patients with left-ventricular dysfunction: the CAPRICORN randomised trial. *Lancet* 2001;357:1385-1390.

16. Yusuf S, Zhao F, Mehta SR, et al: Effects of clopidogrel in addition to aspirin in patients with acute coronary syndromes without ST-segment elevation. *N Engl J Med* 2001;345:494-502.

17. de Winter RJ, Windhausen F, Cornel JH, et al: Early invasive versus selectively invasive management for acute coronary syndromes. *N Engl J Med* 2005;353:1095-1104.

Chapter **6**

Risk Stratification Following Acute Myocardial Infarction

Evaluation of prognosis by systematic risk stratification after acute myocardial infarction (AMI) is fundamental to optimal patient management. It provides an estimate of the probability of long-term survival and recurrent coronary events. It is also essential for the rational selection of patients for coronary angiography and myocardial revascularization. Risk stratification is achieved by a comprehensive evaluation, which entails clinical assessment and objective cardiac tests.[1,2] This process begins with clinical assessment at the time of the patient's admission and is completed by further testing before, or shortly after, hospital discharge. Patients with complicated MI and clinical instability are candidates for direct coronary angiography and potential myocardial revascularization. This chapter pertains only to clinically stable patients.

The specific goals of prognostic assessment in stable post-MI patients are (1) identification of those who are at high or intermediate risk for recurrent coronary events and who may be candidates for myocardial revascularization and (2) identification of those who are at low risk and do not require invasive intervention and management. It is important to emphasize that all post-MI patients should receive comprehensive secondary prevention. The increasing array of cardioprotective drug therapies and lifestyle changes as well as revascularization in appropriate patients, have significantly improved long-term survival after MI (see Chapter 11).

Heterogeneity of Risk in Post-MI Patients

Patients with coronary heart disease (CHD) comprise a heterogeneous population in terms of disease severity and prognosis, especially those who have survived an AMI. Despite recent improvement in survival following MI, these patients remain at increased risk for recurrent coronary events (Figure 6-1).[3] As noted in studies more than 30 years ago, mortality is highest in the early period following MI and subsequently decreases to a relatively constant rate at 3 to 6 months. After the first year, the average mortality approaches that of patients with stable angina (~5% per year). However, within the entire post-MI population, the spectrum of risk is very broad, with annual mortality ranging from less than 2% to more than 50%. On the basis of these findings, survivors of MI have generally been classified into high-, intermediate-, and low-risk groups. The high-risk group (10% to >50% annual mortality) includes approximately 20% of post-MI patients; intermediate-risk patients (5% to 10% annual mortality) account for approximately 25% of the total; the low-risk group (<5% annual mortality) comprises 40% of survivors; and very-low-risk patients (<2% annual mortality) include 15% of the total. This pattern persists into the current era, with contributions from several countervailing mortality trends. Thus, short-term and long-term mortality have fallen because of therapeutic advances and detection of a higher number of small MIs by increasingly sensitive diagnostic methods (eg, serum troponins); by contrast, mortality after MI is considerably elevated in the growing elderly population.

Prognostic Factors

For more than 4 decades, multiple determinants of short-term and long-term prognosis have been identified

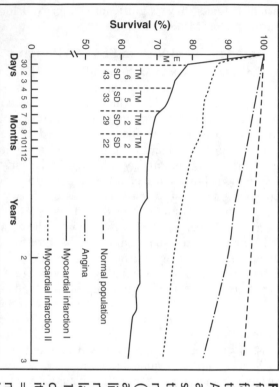

Figure 6-1: Actuarial survival curves for patients with myocardial infarction (MI). The solid line depicts the survival of 1,420 patients with AMI (I) studied between 1979 and 1984, and the dotted line shows the survival of 1,266 patients (II) followed between sex-matched normal population (dashed line) and patients with angina pectoris (dashed/dotted line). The survival rates in the normal population and angina population were significantly higher at 1, 2, and 3 years. EM = early (30-day) mortality; TM = total mortality (percent) for time interval; SD = sudden death (percent of total mortality) for time intervals during the first year after AMI. With permission from Henning H: Prognosis of acute myocardial infarction. In: Francis GS, Alpert JS, eds. *Coronary Care*, 2nd ed. Philadelphia, Lippincott Williams & Wilkins, 1995, pp 689-740.[3]

134

in survivors of AMI. Initial studies of prognosis were based primarily on clinical factors, such as history, physical examination, electrocardiogram (ECG), and radiography. In subsequent investigations, clinical assessment has been complemented by objective data obtained from exercise testing, echocardiography, scintigraphy, and cardiac rhythm monitoring for quantitative evaluation of myocardial ischemia, ventricular function, and arrhythmias. Prognostic evaluation is readily achievable and clinically essential for optimal patient management.

Predictors of short-term and long-term prognosis are evident at the time of admission based on the history, physical examination, ECG, chest radiograph, and serum cardiac injury markers. Estimates of prognosis from these data can be refined by further evaluation with the aforementioned cardiac tests. This approach applies to patients treated with intravenous thrombolytic agents, although proponents of the 'open artery hypothesis' (see below) advocate definitive angiography to assess coronary anatomy in this group. Patients who receive coronary reperfusion therapy by primary angioplasty will already have had coronary angiography and left ventriculography as part of their initial management. Therefore, further prognostic testing is usually limited in this group.

Killip Classification

Because of its simplicity and utility for prognosis in populations of patients with AMI, this method, published in 1967,[4] is still widely employed. The classes are based on clinical assessment (primarily the physical examination) and range from absence of heart failure to cardiogenic shock (Table 6-1). However, clinical assessment alone fails to detect significant cardiac dysfunction in 15% to 20% of patients, and more precise evaluation is provded by quantitative hemodynamic measurement with the Swan-Ganz catheter. This method has shown that early mortality is increased up to 5-fold with left ventricular filling pressure >20 mm Hg and cardiac index <2.0l/min/m^2.[5]

Table 6-1: Classification of Patients With Acute Myocardial Infarction

Killip Class	Criteria	30-day Mortality
I	No CHF	<5%
II	Basilar rales	15%
III	Pulmonary edema	30%
IV	Cardiogenic shock	80%

CHF = congestive heart failure

Patients can be immediately divided into broad categories of risk based on the ECG alone. This simple, inexpensive method can distinguish the site and extent of injury and the culprit coronary artery. The ECG remains the primary tool for identifying candidates for emergency coronary reperfusion therapy because ST elevation is typically related to total thrombotic coronary artery occlusion while the absence of this finding strongly suggests that a coronary thrombosis is not totally occlusive. As discussed in Chapter 5 and shown in Figure 5-6, prognosis can be related to the specific alterations in the ST segment. Acute coronary syndromes (ACS) associated with anterior ST elevation or depression are usually related to occlusion of the left anterior descending coronary artery, which results in more extensive cardiac damage, complications, and mortality than inferior MIs, which are typically caused by occlusion of the right coronary artery. Intermediate degrees of injury are associated with left circumflex coronary artery occlusion, which usually causes lateral wall MI. Additionally, new left bundle-branch block identifies a very high risk group of AMI patients. It is also important to note that approximately 5% of patients with ACS have normal ECGs, which indicates relatively low clinical risk.

Serum Markers of Cardiac Injury and Inflammation

Release of intracellular macromolecules from injured myocytes affords both diagnostic information and an estimate of the extent of myocardial damage. Because factors such as metabolism, binding, excretion, and 'flushing' from the infarct zone by reperfusion therapy influence the blood level of a cardiac marker, this method is more applicable to populations of MI patients than to individuals. Early studies of this approach revealed that markedly elevated plasma levels ($\geq$2,000 IU) of creatine kinase (CK) are associated with a poor prognosis and an increased occurrence of left ventricular failure.

Because of their superior sensitivity and specificity, the cardiac troponins (I and T) are the current standard markers for the diagnosis of AMI. As indicated in Figure 6-2, part A, there is a direct relationship between the blood level of cardiac troponin I and 6-week mortality in patients with non-ST-elevation ACS.[6] Even a small elevation is associated with increased mortality. Further, the troponins have demonstrated superior prognostic value to CK or its MB (myocardial) band. Figure 6-2, part B, which compares the relationship of CK-MB and troponin I with mortality in patients with non-ST-elevation ACS, indicates that cardiac troponin can discriminate between high- and low-risk patients, even within the group with negative CK-MB values.[6]

Current interest in markers of inflammation and CHD risk is considerable. In the TIMI IIA trial of patients with non-ST-elevation ACS, C-reactive protein (CRP) provided prognostic information that was independent of and complementary to that of cardiac troponin T. C-reactive protein identified patients at high risk for short-term mortality even in the group with negative troponin.[7] Additionally, CRP provided independent prognostic information in the PROVE-IT trial of patients with non-ST-elevation ACS.[8]

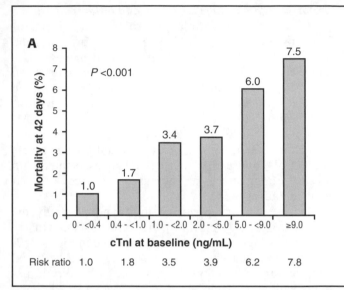

Figure 6-2: Thrombolysis in Myocardial Infarction (TIMI) IIIB. A: A direct relationship was observed between increasing levels of troponin I and a higher 42-day mortality. B: The relationship of positive versus negative troponin I in relation to 42-day mortality in the total group (left) and those with negative creatine kinase (CK)-MB

Noninvasive Cardiac Evaluation

Noninvasive cardiac studies confirmed that post-MI prognosis is closely related to three factors: left ventricular function, myocardial ischemia, and electric instability. Left ventricular function, which is considered the single most important determinant, is readily obtained by measuring left ventricular ejection fraction (LVEF), usually by echocardiography. Myocardial ischemia and electric instability are assessed by cardiac stress testing and rhythm monitoring, respectively. The significance of each of these variables is modified by the clinical and

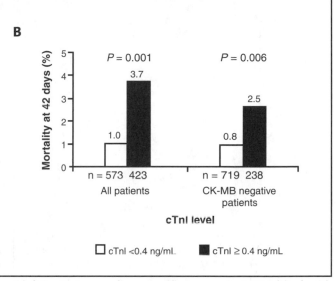

B

(right). cTnI = cardiac-specific troponin I. Modified with permission from Cannon C, Braunwald E: Chapter 10. Unstable angina. In: Braunwald E, Zipes D, Libby P, eds. *Heart Disease,* 6th ed. Philadelphia, WB Saunders, 2001, and adapted with permission from Antman et al, *N Engl J Med* 1996;335:1342-1349.[6]

demographic factors described in the preceding clinical predictive models.

Left ventricular function

Although there may be some restoration of ventricular function by recovery of stunned myocardium after MI, LVEF measured in the peri-MI phase approximates that determined in most patients during the year following discharge. However, detection of viable, ischemic myocardium is an important objective of stress testing. The close, inverse relationship between LVEF and post-MI mortality is a fundamental finding in survivors of MI, as demonstrated

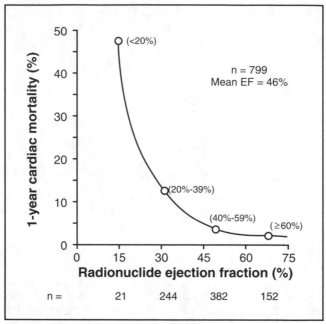

Figure 6-3: Cardiac mortality rate in four categories of radionuclide ejection fraction (EF) determined before discharge (n denotes the number of patients in the total population and in each category). Of 811 patients in whom the EF was recorded, 12 were lost to follow-up during the first year after hospitalization. With permission from *N Engl J Med* 1983;309:331-336.[9]

in Figure 6-3, based on almost 900 patients from the Multi-center Postinfarction Research Group.[9] One-year mortality is relatively low in patients with normal LVEF and rises sharply as radionuclide ejection fraction falls below 40%; with LVEF less than 30%, mortality increases fivefold. This relationship, based on data primarily from the prethrombolytic period, was confirmed in the thrombolytic era by results from the Gruppo Italiano per lo Studio della

Sopravvivenza nell'Infarto Miocardico (GISSI-2) thrombolysis trial obtained by echocardiography.[10] Studies of the
comparative prognostic value of LVEF indicate that it is
superior to other variables, including the history, physical
examination, ECG, and cardiac serum enzyme data, as well
as clinical prognostic indices. Because it is so powerful a
predictor of prognosis, it is recommended that LVEF be
measured in all MI patients before hospital discharge.

Exercise testing and stress imaging

The safety and utility of early post-MI treadmill exercise testing for risk stratification was established more than
20 years ago. The standard test employs a submaximal
stress (treadmill or bicycle) based on variable end points,
including 70% to 80% of age-predicted maximum heart
rate, 5 to 6 METs (multiples of resting oxygen consumption), or absolute heart rate less than 130 beats/minute. In
addition to identification of high-risk patients by ischemic
ST-segment depression, factors associated with poor prognosis during submaximal testing include inability to perform or complete the test, impaired blood pressure response, ventricular tachycardia, and angina. As indicated
in Figure 6-4 from the TIMI II thrombolysis trial, mortality at 52 weeks was lowest in post-MI patients able to
complete a low-level exercise test and highest in those
unable to perform the test.[11] All patients in this study received thrombolytic therapy, and the gradations between
posthospital mortality and exercise test results are similar
to those found in reports from the prethrombolytic era.

Because post-MI outcomes are related to residual ischemia and LVEF, stress imaging studies, which can measure both variables, have excellent predictive results,
which exceed the results of exercise testing and even coronary angiography for posthospital clinical course. In one
study, multivariate analysis revealed that LVEF and residual ischemia were the best predictors of hard events
(death, recurrent MI) and total events (death, MI, unstable
angina, heart failure) and improved risk stratification over

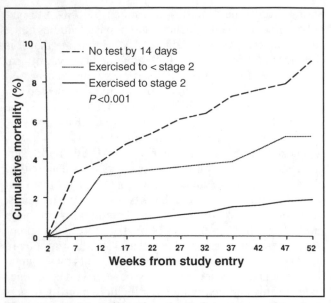

Figure 6-4: Mortality of patients in conservative strategy who did not perform exercise test compared with the mortality of those who were able to complete only one or both stages of low-level predischarge exercise test (*P*<0.001). With permission from Chaitman et al, *Am J Cardiol* 1993;71:131-138.[11]

that of clinical and angiographic data.[12] Echocardiography provides similar quantitation of cardiac variables and risk stratification. In a study of more than 900 post-MI patients evaluated by dipyridamole (Persantine®) echocardiography, a new left ventricular wall motion abnormality indicative of ischemia was the most powerful predictor of subsequent events.[13]

The use of echocardiography to predict functional recovery of regional myocardium in post-MI patients undergoing revascularization was recently extended by analysis of wall motion during exercise. Contractile reserve and a biphasic response (initial improvement of segmental wall motion and subsequent deterioration) of ischemic myocardium during supine exercise echocardiography were the best predictors of recovery of contractile function.[14]

Submaximal treadmill exercise testing provides sufficient data for management of most patients, while a stress-imaging method is indicated in selected patients. These include patients who cannot exercise, patients with baseline ECG abnormalities that preclude interpretation of the exercise ECG, and patients with moderate or severely depressed LVEF in whom the more sensitive stress imaging methods are required.

Ventricular arrhythmias

Ventricular arrhythmias in the peri-MI period, after the first 48 hours, represent persistent electric instability and are predictors of postdischarge mortality. The frequency and complexity (multifocal, runs) of ventricular ectopic beats, detected predischarge by telemetry, ambulatory monitoring, or exercise testing, correlate with late sudden death and total mortality. Patients with severely impaired left ventricular function (ejection fraction <35%) are prone to sudden death, which is reduced by the implantable cardioverter-defibrillator. This finding is the basis for current guidelines recommending the device in such patients, even in the absence of ventricular arrhythmias.[15]

Recent Prognostic Models

To provide a contemporary approach to risk prediction based on current advances, predictive scores have been developed from large clinical trials of patients with ACS.

GUSTO-I

In the GUSTO-I thrombolytic trial of more than 40,000 patients, the prognostic importance of 16 demographic and clinical characteristics was determined by multivariate analysis. A striking finding of this study, as shown in Figure 6-5, is that five variables (age, systolic blood pres-

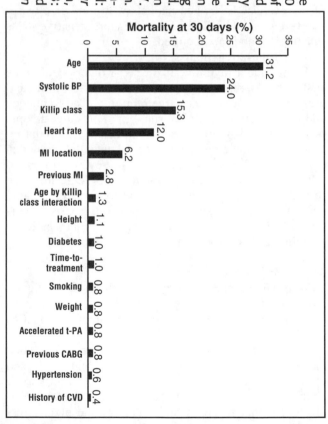

Figure 6-5: A multivariate mode of mortality at 30 days in the Global Use of Strategies to Open Occluded Arteries in Acute Coronary Syndromes (GUSTO-I) trial. The listed factors provide the relative importance in affecting mortality among the 41,021 patients studied. Adapted from Topol EJ, Van de Werf FJ: Chapter 17. Acute myocardial infarction. Early diagnosis and management. In: Topol E, ed: *Textbook of Cardiovascular Medicine.* Philadelphia, Lippincott-Raven, 1998: 395-435, and data adapted from Lee et al, *Circulation* 1995;91:1659-1668.[16]

Mortality at 30 days (%)

Age	31.2
Systolic BP	24.0
Killip class	15.3
Heart rate	12.0
MI location	6.2
Previous MI	2.8
Age by Killip class interaction	1.3
Height	1.1
Diabetes	1.0
Time-to-treatment	1.0
Smoking	0.8
Weight	0.8
Accelerated t-PA	0.8
Previous CABG	0.8
Hypertension	0.6
History of CVD	0.4

sure, Killip class, heart rate, and MI location) accounted for more than 90% of the 30-day mortality.[16] The effect of age on both short-term and long-term post-MI risk has become increasingly important as the growing elderly population contributes a greater proportion of patients to the total MI population. In this regard, it has recently been reported that the recommended tests for post-MI risk stratification arc significantly less likely to be performed in the elderly than in younger patients.[17]

TIMI risk score for NSTEMI

Based on data from more than 5,000 patients in several major trials, the TIMI risk score for UA/NSTEMI is based on seven simple risk factors that can be applied dichotomously to produce a score that predicted 14-day probability of death and ischemic events. The predictor variables were: age ≥65 years, ≥3 coronary artery disease risk factors, prior coronary artery disease (≥50% stenosis), ST-segment deviation on presentation, ≥2 anginal events in the previous 24 hours, aspirin use in the previous 7 days, and elevated serum cardiac markers. The total number of events comprising the end points (all-cause mortality, new or recurrent MI, or urgent revascularization) rose significantly with increasing score (Figure 6-6).[18] In this analysis, it was also shown that the rate of increase in events was lower in patients treated with enoxaparin (Lovenox®) than in patients treated with unfractionated heparin, indicating that the TIMI risk score could be used in therapeutic decision making. It is important to note that this score does not apply to low-risk patients presenting with symptoms suggestive of ACS but abnormal ECG and serum injury markers.

TIMI risk score for STEMI

The TIMI risk score for patients with STEMI is based on analysis of data from the Intravenous tPA for Treatment of Infarcting Myocardium Early II (InTIME II) trial of more than 14,000 patients eligible for thrombolysis.[19] The STEMI score, obtained from the arithmetic sum of eight factors,

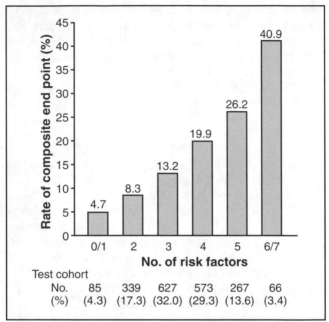

Figure 6-6: Thrombolysis in Myocardial Infarction (TIMI) risk score. Rates of all-cause mortality, myocardial infarction, and severe recurrent ischemia prompting urgent revascularization through 14 days after randomization were calculated for various patient subgroups based on the number of risk factors present in the test cohort (the unfractionated heparin group in the TIMI IIB trial; n =1,957). Event rates increased significantly as the TIMI risk score increased (*P*<0.001 x 2 for trend). With permission from Antman et al, *JAMA* 2000;284:835-842.[18]

predicted 97% of 30-day mortality. A graded difference up to 40-fold was identified by the TIMI score. Mortality was <1% with a score of 0, while a score >8 predicted >35% mortality. The utility of the score was sustained over 1 year.

The Open Artery Hypothesis

The 'open artery hypothesis' refers to the concept that late restoration of patency of the infarct-related coronary artery (IRA) reduces long-term mortality and morbidity after AMI. It has been advanced as a rationale for direct coronary angiography in all post-MI patients to ensure restoration of flow in the IRA by coronary intervention when appropriate. Proposed mechanisms of benefit include limitation of left ventricular remodeling, maintenance of electric stability, and supply of collateral blood flow. Although improved outcomes are supported by some observational studies, there are no controlled trial data on this issue. The largest retrospective analysis of this question (GUSTO-I) revealed that IRA patency was not independently associated with reduced mortality at 1 year.[21] Resolution of this question awaits the results of the Occluded Artery Trial (OAT), a prospective, randomized study that is testing the hypothesis that opening the IRA within 3 to 28 days after AMI in asymptomatic patients with LVEF ≤50% reduces mortality and morbidity over a 3-year follow-up interval.

Summary

The goals of management for survivors of AMI are to prevent mortality and morbidity and to restore each patient to optimal functional status. An algorithm for management is presented in Figure 6-7.[20] It is current practice for most patients who have received thrombolytic therapy to undergo coronary angiography before discharge. Those who receive revascularization by urgent primary coronary intervention have already had coronary angiography. For the remainder of patients, however, as in all aspects of patient care, such algorithms serve as a guideline, and final management decisions require the physician's judgment based on the individual factors in each patient.

Figure 6-7: Algorithm for predischarge management of patients who have had an AMI. It proceeds systematically from assessment by clinical status and left ventricular (LV) function, which determines the noninvasive method for detection of myocardial ischemia. The results of the latter, in turn, provide the basis for selection of medical therapy only or additional evaluation by invasive study (coronary angiography) and possible myocardial revascularization. Patients with persistent or recurrent symptoms of cardiac failure, ischemia, or ventricular arrhythmias (unstable condition) should undergo direct coronary angiography. If anatomy is suitable for revascularization, they are candidates for myocardial revascularization. Deedwania et al, *Arch Intern Med* 1997;157:273-280.[20]

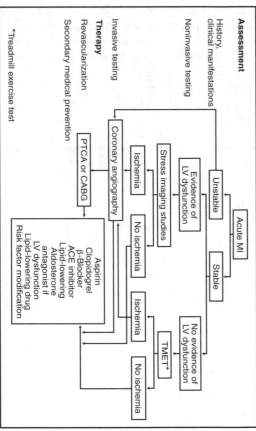

Assessment
History,
clinical manifestations

Noninvasive testing

Invasive testing

Therapy
Revascularization

Secondary medical prevention

*Treadmill exercise test

Acute MI

Unstable

Stable

Evidence of
LV dysfunction

No evidence of
LV dysfunction

Stress imaging studies

Ischemia

No ischemia

TMET*

Ischemia

No ischemia

Coronary angiography

PTCA or CABG

Ischemia

No ischemia

Aspirin
Clopidogrel
β-Blocker
ACE inhibitor
Lipid-lowering
Aldosterone
antagonist if
LV dysfunction
Lipid-lowering drug
Risk factor modification

References

1.   Braunwald E, Antman EM, Beasley JW, et al: ACC/AHA 2002 guideline update for the management of patients with unstable angina and non-ST-segment elevation myocardial infarction—summary article: a report of the American College of Cardiology/American Heart Association task force on practice guidelines (Committee on the Management of Patients With Unstable Angina). *J Am Coll Cardiol* 2002;40:1366-1374.

2.   Antman EM, Anbe DT, Armstrong PW, et al: ACC/AHA guidelines for the management of patients with ST-elevation myocardial infarction: a report of the American College of Cardiology/American Heart Association Task Force on Practice Guidelines (Committee to Revise the 1999 Guidelines for the Management of Patients with Acute Myocardial Infarction). *Circulation* 2004;110:e82-e292.

3.   Francis GS, Alpert JS, eds: *Coronary Care*, 2nd ed, Philadelphia, PA, Lippincott Williams & Wilkins, 1995, pp 663-668.

4.   Killip T 3rd, Kimball JT: Treatment of myocardial infarction in a coronary care unit. A two year experience with 250 patients. *Am J Cardiol* 1967;20:457-464.

5.   Forrester JS, Diamond GA, Swan HJ: Correlative classification of clinical and hemodynamic function after acute myocardial infarction. *Am J Cardiol* 1977;39:137-145.

6.   Antman EM, Tanasijevic MJ, Thompson B, et al: Cardiac-specific troponin I levels to predict the risk of mortality in patients with acute coronary syndromes. *N Engl J Med* 1996;335:1342-1349.

7.   Morrow DA, Rifai N, Antman EM, et al: C-reactive protein is a potent predictor of mortality independently of and in combination with troponin T in acute coronary syndromes: a TIMI 11A substudy. Thrombolysis in Myocardial Infarction. *J Am Coll Cardiol* 1988;31:1460-1465.

8.   Cannon CP, Braunwald E, McCabe CH, et al, for the Pravastatin or Atorvastatin Evaluation and infection Therapy-Thrombolysis in Myocardial Infarction 22 investigators: Intensive versus moderate lipid lowering with statins after acute coronary syndromes. *N Engl J Med* 2004;350:1495-1504.

9.   Risk stratification and survival after myocardial infarction. *N Engl J Med* 1983;309:331-336.

10. Volpi A, De Vita C, Franzosi MG, et al: Determinants of 6-month mortality in survivors of myocardial infarction after throm-

bolysis. Results of the GISSI-2 data base. The Ad hoc Working Group of the Gruppo Italiano per lo Studio della Sopravvivenza nell'Infarto Miocardico (GISSI)-2 Data Base. *Circulation* 1993;88:416-429.

11. Chaitman BR, McMahon RP, Terrin M, et al: Impact of treatment strategy on predischarge exercise test in the Thrombolysis in Myocardial Infarction (TIMI) II Trial. *Am J Cardiol* 1993;71:131-138.

12. Mahmarian JJ: Prediction of myocardium at risk. Clinical significance during acute infarction and in evaluating subsequent prognosis. *Cardiol Clin* 1995;13:355-378.

13. Picano E, Landi P, Bolognese L, et al: Prognostic value of dipyridamole echocardiography early after uncomplicated myocardial infarction: a large-scale, multicenter trial. The EPIC Study Group. *Am J Med* 1993;95:608-618.

14. Lancellotti P, Hoffer EP, Pierard LA: Detection and clinical usefulness of a biphasic response during exercise echocardiography early after myocardial infarction. *J Am Coll Cardiol* 2003;41:1142-1147.

15. Hunt SA: ACC/AHA 2005 guideline update for the diagnosis and management of chronic heart failure in the adult: a report of the American College of Cardiology/American Heart Association Task Force on Practice Guidelines (Writing Committee to Update the 2001 Guidelines for the Evaluation and Management of Heart Failure). *J Am Coll Cardiol* 2005;46:e1-e82.

16. Lee KL, Woodlief LH, Topol EJ, et al: Predictors of 30-day mortality in the era of reperfusion for acute myocardial infarction. Results from an international trial of 41,021 patients. GUSTO-I Investigators. *Circulation* 1995;91:1659-1668.

17. Alexander KP, Galanos AN, Jollis JG, et al: Post-myocardial infarction risk stratification in elderly patients. *Am Heart J* 2001;142:37-42.

18. Antman EM, Cohen M, Bernink PJ, et al: The TIMI risk score for unstable angina/non-ST elevation MI: A method for prognostication and therapeutic decision making. *JAMA* 2000;284:835-842.

19. Morrow DA, Antman EM, Charlesworth A, et al: TIMI risk score for ST-elevation myocardial infarction: A convenient, bedside, clinical score for risk assessment at presentation: An intravenous nPA for treatment of infarcting myocardium early II trial substudy. *Circulation* 2000;102:2031-2037.

20.   Deedwania PC, Amsterdam EA, Vagelos RH: Evidence-based, cost-effective risk stratification and management after myocardial infarction. California Cardiology Working Group on Post-MI Management. *Arch Intern Med* 1997;157:273-280.

21.   Sadanandan S, Buller C, Menon V, et al: The late open artery hypothesis—a decade later. *Am Heart J* 2001;142:411-421.

Chapter **7**

Cardioprotective Drug Therapy

Several pharmacologic agents are now established as standard treatment for secondary prevention of recurrent coronary heart disease (CHD) events in patients who have had an acute myocardial infarction (AMI). Because of their demonstrated efficacy in decreasing long-term CHD morbidity and mortality in randomized clinical trials, these drugs are called 'cardioprotective.' Moreover, they exert their beneficial effects on secondary prevention irrespective of conventional symptomatic indications for their use. They include aspirin, angiotensin-converting enzyme (ACE) inhibitors, and β-blockers and are the major subjects of this chapter. Consideration will also be given to calcium-channel blockers (CCBs), nitrates, and the role of long-term antiarrhythmic modalities. Lipid-lowering drugs are considered in Chapter 4.

Trends in Therapy After Myocardial Infarction

An area of continuing concern in the management of post-MI patients is the inadequate use of proven cardioprotective drug therapy, a phenomenon that has been referred to as the 'knowledge-practice gap.' This problem has been consistently documented in large-scale studies, and, although there has been recent improvement, significant opportunity remains for further gains. National trends in discharge medications for patients after AMI demonstrate that aspirin is the most frequently used drug, followed by β-blockers with increasing use of ACE inhibitors and lipid-lowering agents. In smokers, less than 50% still receive advice on smoking cessation.[1-5]

Aspirin and Other Antiplatelet Agents

Aspirin

The rupture of an atherosclerotic plaque is the initiating process in AMI. Circulating platelets are exposed to thrombogenic factors within the plaque, leading to platelet activation, adhesion, aggregation, and the formation of a flow-limiting thrombus. The efficacy of aspirin as an antiplatelet agent is primarily related to its interference with the biosynthesis of the cyclic prostanoid, thromboxane A_2, a potent platelet activator and vasospastic mediator. Aspirin is the first medication given to patients on presentation to the emergency department for suspected acute coronary syndromes (ACS). The drug is rapidly absorbed from the stomach and reaches appreciable plasma levels in 20 minutes. Platelet inhibition develops in approximately 1 hour. Because of the development of thrombosis as a final pathway for coronary occlusion and resultant AMI, it is rational to administer aspirin as early as possible and to continue its use indefinitely. Pharmacodynamic studies indicate that medium-dose aspirin (162 mg, one half of an adult aspirin) inhibits thromboxane A_2 synthesis and diminishes platelet activity.

Several trials have demonstrated the efficacy of aspirin in modifying short-term and long-term mortality in MI. In the Second International Study of Infarct Survival (ISIS-2), for example, when compared with placebo, 160 mg of aspirin within 24 hours of AMI reduced mortality by 23%, nonfatal reinfarction by 49%, and nonfatal stroke by 46% (Figure 7-1).[6] This trial established the benefit of aspirin in AMI. It has also been demonstrated that aspirin is incrementally beneficial when given in conjunction with thrombolytic agents. Other studies of aspirin initiated early or late after AMI indicate a 5% to 40%

153

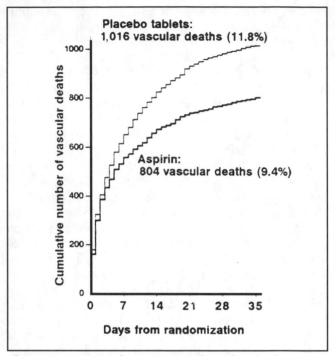

Figure 7-1: Second International Study of Infarct Survival (ISIS-2) results showing all patients allocated active aspirin vs all allocated placebo tablets. Adapted from *Lancet* 1988;2:349-360, with permission.[6]

reduction in cardiac mortality and a 10% to 60% reduction in nonfatal infarction. Nonfatal stroke rate has also been reduced by approximately 40%. A meta-analysis by the Antiplatelet Trialists, comprising 100,000 patients in whom aspirin was used for long-term treatment after AMI and other high-risk cardiovascular conditions, demonstrated a decrease in vascular death of approximately 16% and a decrease in nonfatal MI or stroke of 33%. These results occurred without regard to age, gender, or presence of hypertension or diabetes. Current ACC/AHA guidelines indicate that aspirin should be given indefinitely after MI on a daily basis from 75 mg to 162 mg. Clopidogrel 75 mg/d or warfarin should be considered if aspirin is contraindicated.[7,8]

Warfarin

Several long-term anticoagulant studies have demonstrated efficacy of oral anticoagulants following AMI. For example, in the Warfarin Reinfarction Study (WARIS), warfarin (Coumadin®) decreased mortality by 24% compared with placebo over several years, with decreases of 34% in reinfarction and more than 50% in stroke.[9] Several studies directly comparing aspirin with anticoagulants for long-term postinfarction prophylaxis showed equivalency, although there was a higher frequency of bleeding with the anticoagulants and more frequent gastrointestinal side effects with aspirin.

A recent meta-analysis of the use of warfarin plus aspirin after AMI reviewed 10 trials involving almost 6,000 patients. Warfarin plus aspirin was found to decrease the annual rate of infarction compared with aspirin alone; hazard ratio: 0.56 (95% CI, 0.46 -0.69), although the use of warfarin was associated with an increase in major bleeding HR 2.5 (95% CI, 1.7-3.7).[10] At present, however, as indicated above, warfarin is only indicated by ACC/AHA guidelines as a substitute for aspirin or clopidogrel if the latter two are contraindicated because of side effects not related to bleeding.

Clopidogrel and Ticlopidine

Clopidogrel (Plavix®) and ticlopidine (Ticlid®) are thienopyridine derivatives that inhibit platelet aggregation by a mechanism different from that of aspirin. These drugs block the platelet adenosine diphosphate receptor, which amplifies platelet activation. Clopidogrel does not have the leukopenic side effect of ticlopidine.

Studies of aspirin, ticlopidine, or clopidogrel after AMI have been frequently coupled with thrombolytic therapy.

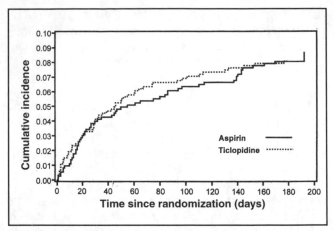

Figure 7-2: Results of the Study of Ticlopidine versus Aspirin After Myocardial Infarction (STAMI) showing lack of difference in cumulative incidence curve for primary end points, aspirin vs ticlopidine. From Scrutinio et al, *J Am Coll Cardiol* 2001;37:1259-1265, with permission.[11]

In one study of ticlopidine vs aspirin after thrombolysis, 6-month follow-up revealed no difference between groups in the combined end points of death, recurrent infarction, stroke, and angina (Figure 7-2).[11]

The Clopidogrel vs Aspirin in Patients at Risk for Ischemic Events trial (CAPRIE) compared aspirin (325 mg/d) with clopidogrel (75 mg/d) for an average of 2 years for prevention of combined events of vascular death, AMI, or stroke in patients with a history of AMI, stroke, or peripheral vascular disease.[12] Event rates were slightly, but significantly, lower with clopidogrel (5.32% vs 5.83% per year, P=0.04), but there was no significant difference in the subset of patients who had a prior AMI. There were no differences in adverse effects. Although there is no evidence that clopidogrel or ticlopidine is more effective than aspirin following ST-elevation

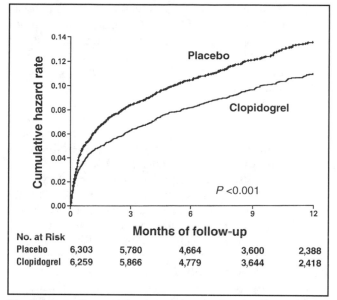

Figure 7-3: Cumulative hazard rates for the first primary outcome (death from cardiovascular causes, nonfatal myocardial infarction, or stroke) during the 12 months of the Clopidogrel in Unstable Angina to Prevent Recurrent Events (CURE) study. Both groups received aspirin. The results demonstrate the sustained effect of clopidogrel. From Yusuf et al, *N Engl J Med* 2001;345: 494-502, with permission.[13]

AMI, the recent Clopidogrel in Unstable Angina to Prevent Recurrent Events (CURE) (Figure 7-3) trial[13] demonstrated the superiority of clopidogrel plus aspirin compared with aspirin alone for long-term treatment of non-ST-elevation ACS. Patients on the two drugs had a 20% reduction (*P*<0.001) of the combined end point of death, recurrent ischemic events, rehospitalization, and revascularization during the 12-month follow-up period after the initial ACS.

A more recent clinical trial involving 45,852 patients admitted with a wide range of AMI indicated that clopidogrel added to aspirin decreased death, reinfarction, or stroke vs placebo in the immediate infarct period (mean of 15 days post-infarct).[14] Another recent study of patients with clinically evident cardiovascular disease or multiple risk factors assigned to clopidogrel plus low-dose aspirin or placebo plus low-dose aspirin suggested a benefit in decreased major cardiovascular events with the drug combination in patients in the subgroup with symptomatic atherothrombosis after a follow-up of 28 months (HR 0.88, 95% CI 0.77-0.998, $P = 0.046$).[15] Clopidogrel remains a secondary agent to be used if aspirin is contraindicated, except after interventional coronary procedures, in which both agents are to be used for up to 1 year, depending on the guideline. Ticlopidine has been largely abandoned because of risk for thrombotic thrombocytopenic purpura or neutropenia.

Platelet Glycoprotein IIb/IIIa Blockers

The final pathway in platelet aggregation is mediated by the glycoprotein (GP) IIb/IIIa receptor, found exclusively on the surface of platelets and megakaryocytes. Through this receptor, fibrinogen combines with platelet aggregates to form the mature red thrombus, which is the culmination of the events initiated by plaque rupture. Platelet GPIIb/IIIa receptor inhibitors have been studied extensively in the treatment of AMI, primarily as adjunctive agents with thrombolysis and coronary angioplasty/stenting in an effort to enhance and sustain reperfusion of the infarct-related artery. There has been limited evaluation of IIb/IIIa receptor inhibitors as isolated treatment after MI. These agents are usually administered for 48 to 72 hours during the acute coronary event. They are available only in intravenously administered forms and, therefore, cannot be used for long-term post-MI therapy.

Combinations of tirofiban (Aggrastat®) with aspirin vs heparin plus aspirin in the acute phase of unstable angina (UA) were shown to favor the IIb/IIIa-aspirin combination in 30-day mortality (2.3% vs 3.6%, $P=0.02$). In the Platelet Receptor Inhibition in Ischemic Syndrome Management in Patients Limited by Unstable Signs and Symptoms (PRISM-PLUS) study of non-ST-elevation ACS, in which all patients received aspirin, tirofiban alone was associated with a higher 30-day mortality than heparin alone at 7 days.[16] However, at 30 days and 6 months, with continued aspirin therapy in each case, early initiation of tirofiban plus heparin produced a better clinical outcome than either agent alone.

In longer studies, combination of a IIb/IIIa inhibitor with aspirin in ACS has produced equivocal results. In a 30-day follow-up study of more than 10,000 patients with non-ST-elevation ACS (Platelet Glycoprotein IIb/IIIa in Unstable Angina: Receptor Suppression Using Integrilin Therapy [PURSUIT] trial) eptifibatide (Integrilin®) administered for up to 72 hours reduced combined fatal and nonfatal MI.[17] Recent meta-analysis of these and other trials of IIb/IIIa receptor antagonists in non-ST-elevation ACS demonstrated a significant decrease in 30-day mortality in patients with diabetes, especially in those undergoing percutaneous coronary interventions.[18,19]

Recent revised guidelines for ST-elevation AMI suggest Class IIb combination pharmacologic reperfusion with the IIb-IIIa inhibitor abciximab and half-dose reteplase or tenecteplase may be considered for prevention of reinfarction in selected patients with anterior MI, age younger than 75 years, and no risk factors for bleeding.[7]

β-Blockers

β-Blockers have multiple properties that appear to have the potential to protect against recurrent myocardial ischemia and infarction. Their antiadrenergic effects lower blood pressure and heart rate, reduce shear stress due to decreased left ventricular (LV) dp/dt, decrease platelet aggregation, and lessen the permeability of the endothelium to atherogenic lipoproteins. Extensive clinical trials over the past 2 decades have demonstrated that β-blockade decreases post-MI mortality and, specifically, sudden cardiac death over several years.[20]

In the β-Blocker Heart Attack Trial (BHAT), 3,837 patients aged 30 to 69 years who had experienced at least one MI were followed up for 2 to 4 years after administration of propranolol (Inderal®) or placebo.[21,22] The trial was stopped 9 months early. During an average 24-month follow-up period, total mortality was 7.2% in the propranolol group and 9.8% in the placebo group. Sudden cardiac death was 3.3% in the propranolol group and 4.6% in the placebo group. Coronary incidence, defined as recurrent nonfatal reinfarction plus fatal CHD, was reduced by 23% in the propranolol group compared with placebo. Based on these results, the investigators concluded that in patients with no contraindications to β-blockers, treatment should be initiated and continued for at least 3 years.

Although BHAT demonstrated efficacy only for high-risk Q-wave MI patients compared with low-risk Q-wave MI patients and showed no significant effect in non-Q-wave MI patients, later studies have shown a beneficial effect even in non-Q-wave MI patients. In this regard, a beneficial effect on sudden cardiac death is not evident with antiplatelet agents. The average reduction in total mortality with β-blockade is approximately 20%, or an absolute decrease from 10% to 8%, while sudden cardiac death is lowered by 32% to 50%.

The major studies demonstrating β-blocker efficacy after AMI include trials of timolol (Blocadren®), propranolol, and metoprolol (Lopressor®, Toprol XL®). These studies were the Norwegian Timolol Trial,[23] the Goteborg Metoprolol Trial,[24] and the Metoprolol in Acute Myocardial Infarction (MIAMI) trial.[25] They show that timolol decreased sudden cardiac death by almost 50%, metoprolol reduced mortality within 24 hours of symptoms by 40%, and propranolol decreased sudden cardiac death by 30%.

Carvedilol (Coreg®), a newer β-blocker with α-blocking properties, has demonstrated potent anti-ischemic, cardioprotective, and antioxidant properties. It has also shown beneficial effects in LV dysfunction. A study of 151 patients with AMI evaluated acute intravenous and long-term (6-month) oral treatment with carvedilol compared with placebo.[26] The number of cardiac events in the carvedilol group was significantly lower than that in the placebo group (18 vs 31). Other improvements in the carvedilol group included greater stroke volume and diastolic filling of the left ventricle.

The recent Carvedilol Post Infarction Survival Control in Left Ventricular Dysfunction (CAPRICORN) trial evaluated 1,959 patients with a proven AMI and LV ejection fraction (LVEF) <40%.[27] Patients were randomized to carvedilol (to a maximum of 25 mg twice daily) or placebo. All patients were taking ACE inhibitors unless intolerant of these agents. Patients with clinical indications for β-blockers were excluded. Although there was no difference in the primary end point of all-cause mortality or hospital admission for cardiovascular problems after a mean of 1.3 years of follow-up, all-cause mortality alone was lower in the carvedilol group (12% vs 15%, $P = 0.03$). Cardiovascular mortality and nonfatal MI were also reduced in patients randomized to carvedilol.

Other end points that showed significant benefit of carvedilol in the CAPRICORN trial included decreases in sudden death (hazard ratio [HR] 0.74), cardiovascular-cause mortality (HR 0.75), nonfatal MI (HR 0.59), and all-cause mortality or nonfatal MI (HR 0.71). The reduction in deaths and recurrent MI was found during both acute and chronic phases of the study. These beneficial outcomes applied equally to patients with objective evidence of LV dysfunction.

CAPRICORN differed from previous β-blocker trials in that the protocol mandated use of ACE inhibitors during the acute phase for at least 48 hours before carvedilol

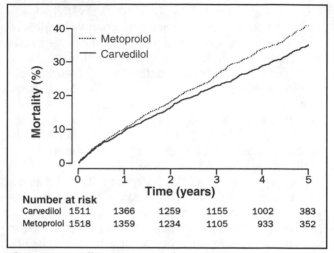

Figure 7-4: All-cause mortality in Carvedilol Or Metoprolol European Trial (COMET). From Poole-Wilson et al, *Lancet* 2003;362:7-13, with permission.[29]

was initiated.[28] This emphasizes the importance of using stable doses of ACE inhibitors as well as diuretics in congestive heart failure patients with AMI before β-blockers are considered.

In the recently published Carvedilol Or Metoprolol European Trial (COMET) in patients with heart failure, carvedilol produced a significantly greater reduction in mortality than metoprolol tartrate.[29] As shown in Figure 7-4, the benefit of carvedilol on mortality occurred early and continued to increase throughout the duration of the trial.[29] COMET is the first head-to-head mortality trial comparing carvedilol, a nonselective β-blocking agent, with metoprolol, a cardioselective β-blocking agent. The multicenter, double-blind study included 3,029 patients with moderate to severe heart failure followed for a mean period of 58 months. The patients were

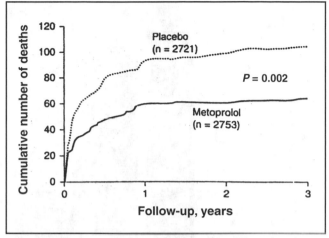

Figure 7-5: Cumulative number of sudden deaths reported in five postinfarction trials. From Kendall et al, *Ann Intern Med* 1995;123:358-367, with permission.[20]

on background therapy with an ACE inhibitor and a diuretic. Although COMET was not a specific post-MI trial, 41% of the patients had a history of MI, and more than 50% had ischemic heart disease.

Pooled data from clinical trials have indicated that the primary effect of β-blockers on decreased long-term mortality after AMI has been due primarily to the reduction of sudden cardiac death (Figure 7-5).[20] Some investigators have questioned whether the decrease in sudden cardiac death is a class effect of β-blockers or is limited to specific agents. For example, the four agents in the major studies described above are lipophilic. Hydrophilic agents such as atenolol (Tenormin®) and sotalol (Betapace®, Betapace AF™) have not shown long-term prophylactic properties in regard to sudden cardiac death.

Despite strong evidence that they provide cardioprotection after AMI, β-blockers have been markedly under-

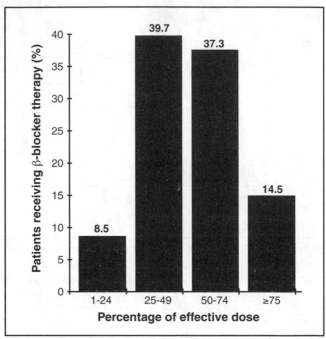

Figure 7-6: Distribution of infarct survivors with relative contraindications to β-blockers who received β-blocker therapy (n=362), according to the dose prescribed at hospital discharge. Dosages of β-blockers are shown as a percentage of effective dosage. From Barron et al, *Prev Cardiol* 1998;3:13-15, with permission.[31]

used in this country, with less than 50% of patients receiving these drugs, according to surveys performed as late as the mid-1990s. The recent incremental increase in β-blocker therapy in post-MI patients may be related partly to the active promotion of this class of drugs through practice guidelines. In addition, the Cardiac Arrhythmia Suppression Trial (CAST),[30] which revealed the adverse effects of antiarrhythmic agents used for long-term

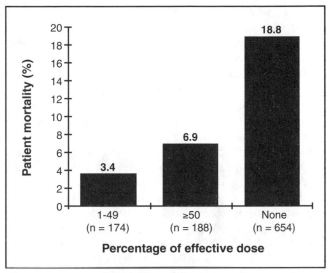

Figure 7-7: Unadjusted long-term mortality rates in patients with relative contraindications to β-blockers who survived the index hospitalization, according to the dose of β-blocker prescribed at hospital discharge. From Barron et al, *Prev Cardiol* 1998;3:13-15, with permission.[31]

prophylaxis after MI, increased awareness of the benefits of β-blockers.

Part of the reluctance of physicians to use β-blockers is attributable to their *relative* contraindications, which include obstructive pulmonary disease, diabetes, and peripheral vascular disease. However, it is now recognized that patients in these groups are at high risk for coronary events, that many can tolerate β-blockers, and that they benefit from β-blockers as much as or more than other patients (Figures 7-6 and 7-7).[31] Patients with compensated pulmonary disease should be given a trial of low-dose β-blocker therapy, which can be continued or increased according to tolerance. In patients with pulmonary disease and non-Q-wave MI, β-blocker therapy has reduced mortality significantly, based on recent clinical trial data. Patients with diabetes appear to have a more beneficial response in terms of decreased mortality compared with patients without diabetes.[32] Clinical trials in post-MI patients with peripheral vascular disease have shown no increase in adverse effects on the latter condition in those on β-blocker therapy compared with placebo. In contrast to the former concern about the use of β-blockers in patients with LV dysfunction, these drugs are now a mainstay in the management of heart failure when used judiciously with other established therapy. Recent clinical trials in congestive heart failure from ischemic and nonischemic cardiomyopathy have shown that β-blockers provide additional benefits of improving survival and LV function. Current guidelines indicate that β-blockers should be started in all patients with AMI and continued indefinitely.[7,8]

Angiotensin-converting Enzyme Inhibitors

Angiotensin II is a potent factor in the pathophysiology of atherosclerosis and coronary ischemic events. Acting through multiple pathways, this peptide exerts proinflammatory, prothrombotic, and atherogenic effects. The beneficial actions of ACE inhibitors are the result of inhibition of converting enzyme activity, reducing both production of angiotensin II and breakdown of bradykinin. These results provide ample protective mechanisms for ACE inhibitors, including decreased oxidative stress, improved fibrinolytic balance, reduced platelet activity, and lower plasminogen activator inhibitor levels. Angiotensin-converting enzyme inhibitors also decrease the migration of macrophages, reduce proliferation of vascular smooth muscle, reduce MI size, and retard detrimental LV remodeling. The beneficial effects of bradykinin include vasodilator actions and protective effects on vascular endothelium (Figure 7-8).[33] The latter are mediated through an

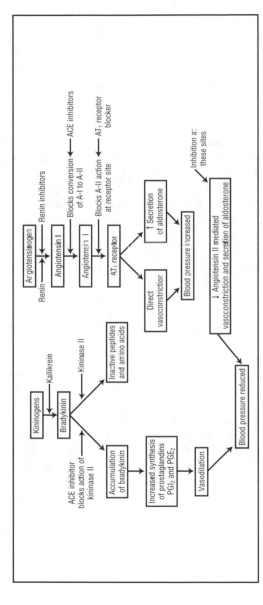

Figure 7-8: Sites of action of various agents on the renin-angiotensin system. Inhibition of kinase activity by angiotensin-converting enzyme (ACE) inhibition allows accumulation of vasodilator substances and contributes to blood pressure lowering. Angiotensin II (A-II) receptor blockade does not affect this system. A-I = angiotensin I, an inactive peptide; AT$_1$ = A-II receptor subtype I; PGE$_2$ = prostaglandin E$_2$; PGI$_2$ = prostacyclin. From Moser, *J Am Coll Cardiol* 1997;29:1414-1421, with permission.[33]

167

increase in nitric oxide (NO) production. In the past decade, the value of ACE inhibitors after AMI has expanded from attenuation of LV remodeling to increased survival and decreased morbidity. Multitrial analysis of early use of ACE inhibitors in more than 100,000 patients (0 to 36 hours from onset of AMI) demonstrates a reduction of 20% to 30% in mortality over 30 days, 80% of which was achieved in the first week of treatment.[34]

The effects of acute intervention with ACE inhibitor therapy during thrombolysis in patients with anterior MI were assessed in the Captopril and Thrombolysis Study (CATS).[35] Captopril (Capoten®) 6.25 mg or placebo was administered to 298 patients immediately on completion of intravenous streptokinase (Streptase®). The captopril dose was repeated at 4 and 8 hours and increased to 12.5 mg and 25 mg at 16 and 24 hours, respectively. The target dose was 25 mg t.i.d. At 1 year, there was less LV dilatation and heart failure in the group with combined thrombolysis and captopril than in the thrombolysis-placebo patients (Figure 7-9). It was concluded that very early ACE inhibitor therapy reduced the occurrence of LV dilatation and progression to heart failure.

Three major studies assessed the effects of ACE inhibitors early (3 to 16 days) after AMI in patients with LV dysfunction or heart failure: Survival and Ventricular Enlargement (SAVE),[36] Acute Infarction Ramipril Efficacy (AIRE),[37] and Trandolapril Cardiac Evaluation (TRACE).[38] Follow-up ranged from 15 months (AIRE) to 50 months (TRACE). The ACE inhibitors were added to diuretics. Mortality was reduced significantly in all three studies: 18% in TRACE, 19% in SAVE, and 27% in AIRE. In AIRE, 2,006 patients were randomized to ramipril (Altace®) or placebo on days 3 to 10 after AMI. Ramipril reduced the risk of sudden cardiac death by 30%, and the decrease in mortality was apparent at 30 days.

After an average follow-up of 15 months, in addition to the 27% ($P<0.002$) decrease in all-cause mortality,

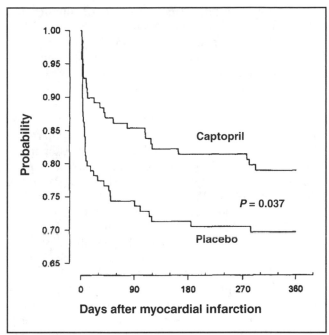

Figure 7-9: Curves representing the absence of heart failure during 1-year follow-up period for captopril-treated patients compared with the placebo group in the Captopril and Thrombolysis Study (CATS). From van Gilst et al, *J Am Coll Cardiol* 1996;28:114-121, with permission.[35]

ramipril produced a 19% ($P<0.008$) reduction in the prespecified end points of cardiac death, heart failure, and stroke. There was no difference in medication withdrawals in the ramipril and placebo groups. A long-term evaluation (42 to 59 months) following the initial AIRE results demonstrated a relative risk reduction of 36% in all-cause mortality (absolute reduction, 11%) in the ACE inhibitor group.[39]

SAVE evaluated the effects of captopril administered to 2,231 patients 3 to 16 days after AMI with LV dysfunction.[36] The initial dose of captopril, 12.5 mg, was progressively increased to a target of 50 mg t.i.d. and compared with placebo. The beneficial effects of captopril included attenuating hemodynamic dysfunction and ventricular dilatation after 1 year. These results were paralleled in the captopril patients by significantly improved clinical outcomes, including reduced cardiovascular mortality and multiple cardiovascular end points. After an average follow-up of 42 months, captopril reduced mortality by 19% ($P<0.02$), new heart failure by 37% ($P<0.001$), and recurrent MI by 25% ($P<0.01$).

TRACE included 1,749 patients randomized to trandolapril (Mavik®), (up to 4 mg/day) or placebo 3 to 7 days after AMI with LV dysfunction.[38] Echocardiographically estimated LV ejection fraction ≤35% was an inclusion criterion. There was a significant increase in survival in patients on trandolapril compared with placebo: 6.2 years vs 4.6 years post-MI, respectively (+27 months, 95% confidence interval 7 to 51). It was also noted that the number of lives saved after 1, 2, and 4 years was 32, 55, and 66 per 1,000 patients treated, respectively.

The composite result of these three trials was a reduction in overall mortality of approximately 20% by ACE inhibitors, with the number of lives saved ranging from 40 to 70 per 1,000 patients treated.[40] A meta-analysis of 15 trials of ACE inhibitor therapy after MI, including more than 15,000 patients, provided strong evidence for ACE inhibitor reduction of sudden cardiac death.[41]

A relevant question is which ACE inhibitor to choose. It is probably not advisable to choose an agent that has not demonstrated efficacy in clinical trials because the agents in this class have different half-lives and metabolisms. The results of current clinical trials indicate that ACE inhibitors should be started during the acute phase of MI and maintained indefinitely, at least in patients with objective evidence of LV dysfunction, regardless of whether congestive heart failure is present (Table 7-1).[40] However, the results of the Heart Outcomes Prevention Evaluation (HOPE) study provide a basis for considering long-term administration of ACE inhibitors to all patients older than 55 years with coronary artery disease.[42]

The results of the HOPE study have an important bearing on the general application of ACE inhibitors in CHD. The study involved 9,297 high-risk men and women older than 55 years and with evidence of vascular disease (cerebral, coronary, or peripheral) or diabetes (patients with diabetes also had one additional risk factor) but no evidence of heart failure or low LVEF. In one arm of the trial, patients were assigned to receive ramipril or placebo for 5 years with evaluation of the primary outcome of MI, stroke, or death from cardiovascular disease. Administration of ACE inhibitors decreased cardiovascular mortality from 8.6% to 6.1%, MI from 12.3% to 9.9%, and stroke from 4.9% to 3.4%. Cardiac arrest, heart failure, and complications of diabetes were also significantly reduced. These differences occurred despite treatment in both groups that included β-blockers (39%), aspirin or other antiplatelet agents (75% to 77%), and lipid-lowering agents (28%). The beneficial effect of ramipril was similar regardless of patient age, gender, antecedent cardiovascular disease, or prior MI. A striking additional finding was the reduction in new-onset diabetes in the ramipril patients. The results support the use of ACE inhibitors in middle-aged men and women with cardiovascular disease or in those at high risk for CHD. Whether to extrapolate these findings to younger patients in these categories must be determined on an individual patient basis. Comparative data on ACE inhibitors regarding dosage and half-life are shown in Table 7-2.[43]

A recent trial (PEACE) suggests that ACE inhibitors in stable coronary disease do not appear to have any advantage in reducing death from CV causes, nonfatal MI, or coro-

Table 7-1: Summary of Randomized Clinical Trials in High-risk Myocardial Infarction Patients

	SAVE[36]	AIRE[37]	TRACE[38]
Pts randomized	2,231	2,006	1,749
Population	EF ≤40%	CHF	WMI <1.2
Drug initiation from MI (days)	3-16	3-10	3-7
Drug dose (mg)	Cap 12.5 -50 t.i.d.	Ram 2.5 -5 b.i.d.	Tran 1-4
Follow-up (mo)	24-60	6-30	24-50
Mortality (%)			
Control	24.6	23	62.3
Treated	20.4	17	34.7
Reduction (%)	19	27	18
P	0.019	0.002	0.001
Lives saved/ 1,000/month	1.0	3.5	2.9

EF = ejection fraction; MI = myocardial infarction;
CHF = congestive heart failure; WMI = wall motion index;
Cap = captopril (Capoten®); Ram = ramipril (Altace®);
Zof = zofenopril;
Enal = enalapril (Vasotec®); Tran= trandolapril (Mavik®)

nary revascularization with normal or slightly diminished LV function, especially when patients are otherwise on optimal cardioprotective therapy, such as aspirin, β-blocker, or lipid-lowering agents.[44] However, current secondary prevention guidelines of the American Heart Association based

SMILE[46]	CATS[35]	CONSENSUS II[45]
1,556	298	6,090
Ant MI	Ant MI	MI
Non-T	T	
≤1	≤6 h	≤1
Zof 7.5	Cap 6.25	Enal 5
-30	-25	-20 b.i.d.
12	3	mean 6
6.5	4.0	9.4
4.9	6.0	10.2
24	—	—
0.198	0	0
11.2	—	—

Adapted from Latini et al, *Circulation* 1995;92:3132-3137.[40]

on the HOPE study results recommend consideration of ACE inhibitors for all patients with vascular disease.

Recently, concern has arisen about a possible adverse interaction between aspirin and ACE inhibitors. The pharmacodynamic effects of ACE inhibitors and aspirin on

Table 7-2: Comparative Data on Angiotensin-Converting Enzyme Inhibitors

Drug	Dosing Range (mg)	Target Dose (mg/day)
Benazepril (Lotensin®)	5-40	20
Captopril (Capoten®)	25-50	150
Enalapril (Vasotec®)	5-40	20
Fosinopril (Monopril®)	10-40	20
Lisinopril (Prinivil®, Zestril®)	5-40	20
Moexipril (Univasc®)	7.5-30	15
Perindopril (Aceon®)	4-16	8
Quinapril (Accupril®)	5-80	20
Ramipril (Altace®)	1.25-20	10
Trandolapril (Mavik®)	1-8	4

Adapted from O'Keefe et al, *J Am Coll Cardiol* 2001;37:1-8.[43]

prostaglandin synthesis are counteractive. This may be especially important in moderate to severe heart failure, in which prostaglandin synthesis, inhibited by aspirin, may be an important mechanism of vasodilation, potentially enhanced by ACE inhibitors. The Cooperative New Scandinavian Enalapril Survival Study II (CONSENSUS II) trial evaluated early administration of enalapril (Vasotec®) within 24 hours of MI and did not show improved survival during 180 days of follow-up (Figure 7-10).[45] A follow-up evaluation of that trial indicated excess mortality when enalapril was randomized to patients using aspirin. By contrast, a meta-analysis of all trials involving more than 100,000 patients randomly allocated to ACE inhibitors

Half-life (h)	Available Dosage Forms
10-11	5, 10, 20, 40 mg tabs
<2	12.5, 25, 50, 100 mg tabs
11	2.5, 5, 10, 20 mg tabs; 1.25 mg/mL injection
11	10, 20, 40 mg tabs
13	2.5, 5, 10, 20, 40 mg tabs
2-9	7.5, 15 mg tabs
8-10	2, 4, 8 mg tabs
2	5, 10, 20, 40 mg tabs
13-17	1.25, 2.5, 5, 10 mg tabs
16-24	1, 2, 4 mg tabs

early in AMI and continuing for at least 4 to 6 weeks showed that ACE inhibitor therapy was associated with similar proportional reductions in 30-day mortality compared with controls, regardless of whether aspirin was also administered.[34] These trials included the Chinese Cardiac Study (CCS-1),[47] CONSENSUS II,[45] GISSI-3,[48] and ISIS-4,[49] totaling more than 96,000 patients, of whom 89% received aspirin. Killip class II or III heart failure was present in 17% of patients in the aspirin group and 26% of patients in the no-aspirin group. The results indicate that, in general, aspirin and ACE inhibitors are both beneficial early in MI.

ACE inhibitors increase prostaglandin production by limiting the breakdown of bradykinin, reducing blood pres-

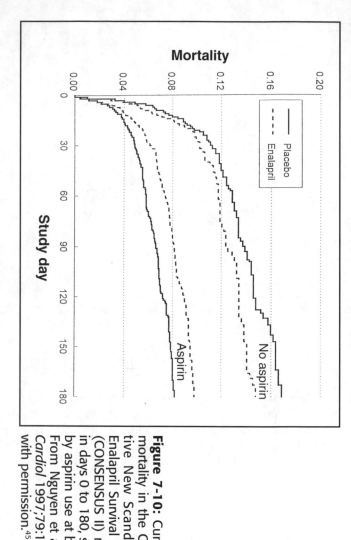

Figure 7-10: Cumulative mortality in the Cooperative New Scandinavian Enalapril Survival Study II (CONSENSUS II) reported in days 0 to 180, stratified by aspirin use at baseline. From Nguyen et al, *Am J Cardiol* 1997;79:115-119, with permission.[45]

sure. Because aspirin inhibits synthesis of prostaglandin I2, it is possible that reduction of blood pressure could be partially inhibited in addition to potentiating depression of renal function by decrease of renal prostaglandin production.

Some retrospective studies also suggest coadministration of aspirin with ACE inhibitors decreases mortality benefit of ACE inhibitors in ischemic heart disease or heart failure, but other studies have not found a decrease in mortality. It has been recommended by some that if aspirin is given with ACE inhibitors, the aspirin dose be confined to 81 mg.

ACE inhibitors are recommended indefinitely for all patients with AMI , with the specification that use is especially indicated for patients with anterior infarction, pulmonary congestion, or LV ejection fraction less than 0.40.[7,8]

Angiotensin II Receptor Blockers

While ACE inhibitors block the effects of angiotensin II by reducing its synthesis, angiotensin II receptor blockers (ARBs) provide more specific antagonism by blocking the angiotensin II AT_1 receptor. These agents have not been tested to the extent of ACE inhibitors for efficacy following AMI, but trials are now under way, and one has been reported. The recently published Optimal Trial in Myocardial Infarction with the Angiotensin II Antagonist Losartan (OPTIMAAL) compared the effects on mortality and morbidity of treatment with losartan (Cozaar®) vs captopril.[50] The trial included more than 5,000 patients with MI and heart failure during the acute phase or a new Q-wave anterior infarction or reinfarction. Losartan was titrated to a target dose of 50 mg once daily, and captopril was titrated to a dose of 50 mg t.i.d., as tolerated. During a mean follow-up interval of 2.7 years, there was a nonsignificant difference in total mortality favoring captopril (18% vs 16%; relative risk 1.13; P=0.07). There were also no significant differences in the secondary and tertiary cardiac end points of mortality and morbidity. However, losartan therapy was better tolerated than captopril. Therefore, this study supports the primary role of ACE inhibitors in the treatment of post-MI LV dysfunction, with consideration of ARBs when ACE inhibitors are not well tolerated. The Valsartan in Acute Myocardial Infarction (VALIANT) trial compared outcomes after AMI associated with LV dysfunction or heart failure in patients treated with captopril, valsartan (Diovan®), or combination therapy with both agents.[51] The 2003 study involved more than 14,000 patients with AMI and is important in demonstrating the noninferiority of an ARB compared with an ACE inhibitor for decreasing cardiovascular events in high-risks patients after MI.

VALIANT randomized patients within 10 days of AMI to valsartan, valsartan plus captopril, or captopril.[51] Over a median follow-up of 2 years, no significant differences were seen for the primary end points of overall mortality and the composite end point of fatal and nonfatal cardiovascular events in the three groups. For the rate of death from any cause, $P=0.98$ for valsartan vs captopril and $P=0.73$ for valsartan + captopril vs captopril. For the rate of death from cardiovascular causes, reinfarction, or hospitalization for heart failure, $P=0.20$ for valsartan vs captopril and $P=0.37$ for valsartan + captopril vs captopril. A statistical assessment of noninferiority was used to evaluate the outcomes, demonstrating the statistical significance of the results. The conclusion of this evaluation was that ARBs appear to be as effective as ACE inhibitors in reducing atherosclerotic events after AMI.

In the OPTIMAAL trial, there had been a strong trend in favor of the ACE inhibitor for death from any cause.[50] However, the ARB dose had not been optimal (losartan 50 mg/d vs captopril 150 mg/day). The VALIANT trial used optimal doses of the ARB (up to 160 mg/day), thus raising the question of whether higher doses would have increased the effectiveness of losartan in OPTIMAAL.

Angiotensin II receptor blockers appear to have equal efficacy to ACE inhibitors in the treatment of hypertension, and early findings suggest that this is also true for congestive heart failure. However, the recently completed Evaluation of Losartan in the Elderly II (ELITE II) trial involving more than 3,000 patients with congestive heart failure demonstrated that the ARB losartan was better tolerated than the ACE inhibitor captopril, although there was no difference in survival.[52] In small-scale studies, combination therapy with ACE inhibitors and ARBs appears to be superior to ACE inhibitor monotherapy in regard to exercise tolerance, hemodynamic effects, and neurohumoral attenuation. The Randomized Evaluation of Strategies for Left Ventricular Dysfunction (RESOLVD) pilot study indicated superiority of combination therapy in preventing LV dilatation and improving LVEF.[53]

Although the combination of an ACE inhibitor and an ARB may be beneficial in the setting of congestive heart failure or decreased LV function in improving symptoms and hemodynamic function, there is no evidence for improved survival with this approach. In general, current guidelines suggest the use of ARBs after AMI in those intolerant to ACE inhibitors and with either clinical or radiologic signs of heart failure or LVEF <0.40. Additionally, eplerenone, a selective aldosterone blocker, has been demonstrated to decrease morbidity and mortality after AMI in patients with LV dysfunction.[54]

Calcium-Channel Blockers

Three types of agents currently make up the CCB group: dihydropyridines, verapamil (Calan®, Covera-HS®, Isoptin®, Verelan®), and diltiazem (Cardizem®, Dilacor®, Tiazac®). There is evidence of an adverse effect of the short-acting form of nifedipine (Adalat®, Procardia®), particularly at high doses, in patients with ACS and chronic CHD. On the other hand, there is no clear evidence for adverse effects of nondihydropyridines instituted after AMI. For example, the Danish Study of Verapamil in Myocardial Infarction (DAVIT I and II) resulted in a trend toward benefit in the verapamil groups.[55] Diltiazem has been extensively evaluated on the basis of the Diltiazem Reinfarction Trial and other multi-institutional studies. Although diltiazem was shown to exert no overall effect on mortality or cardiac events in patients with previous infarction, it was beneficial after non-Q-wave infarctions associated with adequate LV function in preventing severe angina and reinfarction, without effect on mortality. However, mortality was increased in patients with depressed LV function. In the results of the long-term Multicenter Diltiazem Postinfarction trial, with follow-up of 25 months, diltiazem reduced the early (<6 months) but not the late (>6 months) rate of reinfarction.[56]

More recent studies, especially with long-acting CCBs, have shown no adverse effect on mortality or a slight benefit. Long-term follow-up of the previously described clinical trial subjects with non-Q-wave MI on verapamil or diltiazem demonstrated a covariate adjusted decreased risk of 0.69 (95% confidence interval 0.49-0.97) compared with placebo.[57] In a recently published, community-based registry of MI and cardiac death from the World Health Organization Monitoring Trends and Determinants of Cardiovascular Disease (MONICA) Project, involving almost 4,000 patients with nonfatal suspected MI, no excess risk of recurrent MI or death was found in patients receiving nifedipine, verapamil, or diltiazem compared with patients not receiving CCBs or β-blockers.[58]

In summary, long-acting CCBs can be recommended as adjunctive agents for blood pressure control and decrease in anginal symptoms in postinfarction patients whose symptoms are not controlled by standard therapy, especially β-blockers. However, CCBs should not be used for cardioprotection.

Nitrates

Except, possibly, for the use of intravenous nitrates during the early acute infarction period, there is variable evidence that prolonged nitrate administration affects survival. The relevance of nitrates after hospital discharge relates to their effect on decreasing ischemic symptoms and their use as an adjunct to hydralazine (Apresoline®) in patients with significant LV dysfunction when ACE inhibitors and ARBs are contraindicated. Their therapeutic efficacy in chronic use has been considered to be related primarily to venodilatation, resulting in decreased preload and, thereby, reduced myocardial oxygen consumption. More recently, large coronary artery dilation has taken on increasing significance as a mechanism of the anti-ischemic action of nitrates. Large multicenter studies over 4 to 6 weeks following AMI suggest a decrease in cardiac events during that short period. GISSI-3 [48,49] and ISIS-4 [48,49] showed a trend toward overall decrease in cardiac events, although there were no significant effects on cardiac mortality. Because of tolerance to nitrates, a nitrate-free interval is important in their administration. If nitroglycerin patches are used, an 8- to 12-hour drug-free period is necessary. The effective dose varies widely in individual patients. Recommended doses are isosorbide dinitrate 10 to 50 mg q 8 h, transdermal nitroglycerin patch 0.4, 0.8, or 1.2 mg for 12 to 14 hours daily, or isosorbide-5-mononitrate 30 to 120 mg q.d.

Antiarrhythmic Agents

CAST[30] and other relevant studies have demonstrated that the reduction of ventricular ectopy by antiarrhythmic agents may be accompanied by proarrhythmic effects leading to increased mortality and morbidity or, at best, no mortality benefit. Based on these findings, the routine use of antiarrhythmic drugs post-MI is contraindicated. The main concern raised by postinfarction ventricular dysrhythmias is their significance as a

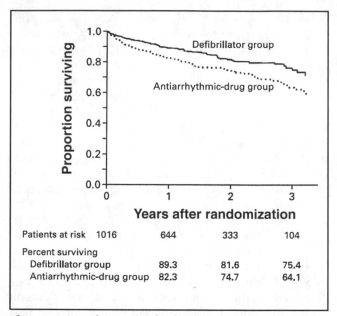

Figure 7-11: The Antiarrhythmics Versus Implantable Defibrillators (AVID) trial. A comparison of antiarrhythmics vs cardioverter-defibrillators in patients resuscitated from near-fatal ventricular fibrillation. Overall survival, unadjusted for baseline characteristics. Survival was better in patients treated with implantable cardioverter-defibrillator ($P<0.02$, adjusted for repeated analyses [n = 6]). From *N Engl J Med* 1997;337:1576-1583, with permission.[60]

risk factor for sudden cardiac death due to ventricular fibrillation. Of the average 3% to 5% posthospital annual mortality after MI, more than 50% is due to sudden death.[59] (The efficacy of β-blockers in decreasing postinfarction mortality, largely by decreasing the incidence of sudden death, has been considered earlier in this chapter.) Predischarge risk for sudden death has been evaluated by several noninvasively obtained criteria, of which the most widely used have been (1) low LVEF, (2) exercise-induced myocardial ischemia, and (3) frequency of ventricular premature depolarizations.[59] More recently, decreased heart rate variability and abnormal signal-averaged electrocardiography (ECG) (late potentials) have been applied to further identify high risk for sudden death. Those at high risk on the basis of these test findings have usually been treated with an implantable cardioverter-defibrillator (ICD) and/or amiodarone (Cordarone®, Pacerone®) (Figure 7-11).[60,61] The order of most sensitive to least sensitive evaluator for serious dysrhythmias is (1) heart rate variability, (2) late potentials, (3) frequent ventricular ectopic beats, and (4) LVEF <40%. Of these, only heart rate variability has a sensitivity >80% (Table 7-3).[62] All four have comparably high specificities. It has been recommended by several authors that, in patients with evidence for ventricular dysrhythmias in the postinfarction state, initial evaluation by signal-averaged ECG and LV ejection be accomplished (Table 7-4).[63] If both tests are positive (ie, positive late potentials are found and LVEF is <40%), the 2-year probability of a serious ventricular dysrhythmia would be >35%, and ICD implantation should be strongly considered. If only one test is positive, ambulatory ECG with a heart rate variability study should be performed. If both of these tests are abnormal (decreased heart rate variability and major ventricular dysrhythmias on ambulatory ECG), ICD implantation should be considered. If only one of these studies is abnormal, electrophysiologic testing for vulnerability to life-threatening ventricular dysrhythmias should be performed. This is only one of a number of possible risk stratification pathways. Repetition of this risk stratification can be accomplished at times beyond hospitalization if further evidence of ventricular electrophysiologic instability arises.

Table 7-3: Comparison of Holter Variables, Late Potentials, Ejection Fraction, and Exercise Test in the Prediction of Arrhythmic Events After Myocardial Infarction

	Sensitivity (%)
Heart rate variability <20 msec	92
Mean relative risk interval <750 msec	67
Late potentials	63
Ventricular ectopic beats <10/h	54
Repetitive ventricular forms	54
Ejection fraction <40%	46
Positive exercise test	50

From Farrell et al, *J Am Coll Cardiol* 1991;18:687-697, with permission.[62]

There is compelling evidence from the recently published Multicenter Automatic Defibrillator Implantation Trial II (MADIT II) (Figure 7-12),[64] together with previous trials, that ICDs improve survival over anti-arrhythmic therapy, usually amiodarone, in post-MI patients at high risk for sudden death. High risk in these studies is usually identified by prior MI, reduced LV function (LVEF <30%), and ambient high-grade ventricular ectopy (ie, nonsustained ventricular tachycardia). In this setting, ICD implantation has become the therapy of choice.

Hormone Replacement Therapy

Hormone replacement with estrogens and progestins in postmenopausal women has been shown to be associ-

Specificity (%)	Positive Predictive Accuracy (%)	Negative Predictive Accuracy (%)
77	17	77
72	13	97
81	17	81
82	16	82
81	15	97
75	10	75
50	6	50

ated with adverse events in secondary prevention after AMI and should not be started at the time of AMI.[65]

Conclusions

Based on the considerations discussed and the guidelines for management of patients after AMI to prevent cardiac mortality, morbidity, and progression of LV dysfunction, the following recommendations are made for patients leaving the hospital after AMI. Antiplatelet agents, β-blockers, and ACE inhibitors should be administered indefinitely. Antiplatelet dosage should be targeted at 75 to 325 mg/d for aspirin. If aspirin is contraindicated, consider clopidogrel 75 mg/d or warfarin. The international normalized ratio should be kept in the range of 2.0 to 3.0 IU for the latter. Angiotensin-converting enzyme inhibitor dosage

Table 7-4: Comparison of Tests for Predicting Major Arrhythmic Events After Myocardial Infarction

Test (No. of Reports)	Number of Patients Studied	Prior Probability (ie, Total MAE Incidence) (Annualized)
ECG-based Tests		
SAECG (22)	9,883	7.99% (4.1%)
SVA (16)	9,564	6.50% (3.33%)
HRV (11)	5,719	9.02% (4.72%)
Left Ventricular Function		
LVEF	7,294	8.57% (4.41%)
Electrophysiologic Studies		
EPS (9)	4,022	8.11% (4.17%)

CI = confidence interval; ECG = electrocardiography; EPS = electrophysiologic study; FN = false negative; FP = false positive; HRV = heart rate variability; LVEF = left ventricular ejection fraction; MAE = major arrhythmic events; SAECG = signal-averaged electro-

Composite Weighted Values for:		2-Year Probability of an MAE if:		Relative Risk	Odds Ratio
Sensitivity (95% CI)	Specificity (95% CI)	Test (+) (95% CI)	Test (-) (95% CI)	(Test +/ Test -)	[(TP/FP)/ (FN/TN)]
62.4% (56.4%-67.9%)	77.4% (73.6%-80.8%)	19.3% (18.3%-20.3%)	4.05% (3.65%-4.48%)	4.8	5.7
42.8% (32.7%-53.7%)	80.9% (75.0%-85.7%)	13.4% (13.0%-13.7%)	4.68% (4.12%-5.18%)	2.9	3.2
49.8% (37.5%-62.1%)	85.8% (82.1%-88.9%)	25.8% (25.0%-25.6%)	5.48% (4.37%-6.52%)	4.7	6.3
59.1% (53.3%-64.6%)	77.8% (75.5%-79.9%)	20.0% (19.8%-19.9%)	4.70% (4.21%-5.19%)	4.3	5.1
61.6% (48.2%-73.4%)	84.1% (65.0%-93.8%)	25.5% (15.6%-40.7%)	3.88% (3.49%-4.65%)	6.6	8.5

cardiography; SVA = serious ventricular arrhythmia; TN = true negative; TP = true positive.

From Bailey et al, *J Am Coll Cardiol*, 2001;38:1902-1911, with permission.[63]

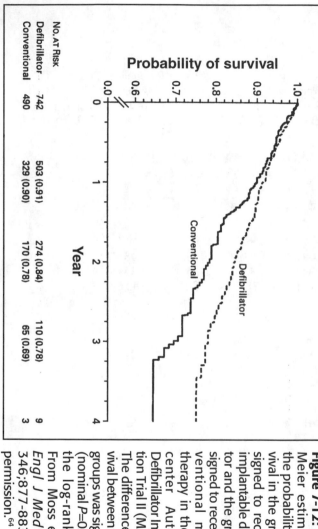

Figure 7-12: Kaplan-Meier estimates of the probability of survival in the group assigned to receive an implantable defibrillator and the group assigned to receive conventional medical therapy in the Multicenter Automatic Defibrillator Implantation Trial II (MADIT II). The difference in survival between the two groups was significant (nominal P=0.007, by the log-rank test). From Moss et al, *N Engl J Med* 2002; 346:877-883, with permission.[64]

should be gradually increased to achieve (1) evidence of LV afterload reduction by lowering systolic blood pressure to <120 mm Hg or (2) a maximum tolerated dose. β-blockers should be administered in optimal dosage, based on the resting heart rate. It would be advisable to reduce heart rate to <75 beats/minute at rest. Long-acting CCBs may be considered for adjunctive therapy for hypertension if β-blockers and ACE inhibitors do not achieve goal blood pressure. Nitrates are not indicated in patients without angina, but patients should always carry a short-acting nitrate to use if needed. Antiarrhythmic agents are not indicated after uncomplicated MI, but asymptomatic patients at risk for lethal arrhythmias should be considered for an ICD. Once-daily medication will increase patient compliance.

References

1.   Rogers WJ, Canto JG, Lambrew CT, et al: Temporal trends in the treatment of over 1.5 million patients with myocardial infarction in the US from 1990 through 1999: the National Registry of Myocardial Infarction 1, 2, and 3. *J Am Coll Cardiol* 2000;36:2056-2063.

2.   Fonarow GC, French WJ, Parsons LS, et al: Use of lipid-lowering medications at discharge in patients with acute myocardial infarction: data from the National Registry of Myocardial Infarction 3. *Circulation* 2001;103:38-44.

3.   Heidenreich PA, McClellan M: Trends in treatment and outcomes for acute myocardial infarction: 1975-1995. *Am J Med* 2001; 110:165-174.

4.   Burwen DR, Galusha DH, Lewis JM, et al: National and state trends in quality of care for acute myocardial infarction between 1994-1995 and 1998-1999: the medicare health care quality improvement program. *Arch Intern Med* 2003;163:1430-1439.

5.   Vaccarino V, Rathore SS, Wenger NK, et al: Sex and racial differences in the management of acute myocardial infarction, 1994 through 2002. *N Engl J Med* 2005;353:671-682.

6.   ISIS-2 Collaborative Group: Randomised trial of intravenous streptokinase, oral aspirin, both or neither among 17,187 cases of suspected acute myocardial infarction. Second International Study of Infarct Survival. *Lancet* 1988;2:349-360.

7. Antman EM, Anbe DT, Armstrong PW, et al: ACC/AHA Guidelines for the management of patients with ST-elevation myocardial infarction—executive summary: a report of the American College of Cardiology/American Heart Association Task Force on Practice Guidelines (Writing Committee to Revise the 1999 Guidelines for the Management of Patients With Acute Myocardial Infarction). *Circulation* 2004;110:588-606.

8. Braunwald E, Antman EM, Beasley JW, et al: ACC/AHA 2002 guideline update for the management of patients with unstable angina and non-ST-segment elevation myocardial infarction: a report of the American College of Cardiology/American Heart Association Task Force on Practice Guidelines (Committee on the Management of Patients With Unstable Angina). *J Am Coll Cardiol* 2002;40:1366-1374.

9. Smith P, Arnesen H, Holme I: The effect of warfarin on mortality and reinfarction after myocardial infarction. *N Engl J Med* 1990;323:147-152.

10. Rothberg MB, Celestin C, Fiore LD, et al: Warfarin plus aspirin after myocardial infarction or the acute coronary syndrome: meta-analysis with estimates of risk and benefit. *Ann Intern Med* 2005;143:241-250.

11. Scrutinio D, Cimminiello C, Marubini E, et al: Ticlopidine versus aspirin after myocardial infarction (STAMI) trial. *J Am Coll Cardiol* 2001;37:1259-1265.

12. CAPRIE Steering Committee: A randomised, blinded, trial of clopidogrel versus aspirin in patients at risk of ischaemic events (CAPRIE). *Lancet* 1996;348:1329-1339.

13. Yusuf S, Zhao F, Mehta SR, et al: Effects of clopidogrel in addition to aspirin in patients with acute coronary syndromes without ST-segment elevation. *N Engl J Med* 2001;345:494-502.

14. Chen ZM, Jiang LX, Chen YP, et al, COMMIT (Clopidogrel and Metoprolol in Myocardial Infarction Trial) collaborative group: Addition of clopidogrel to aspirin in 45,852 patients with acute myocardial infarction: randomised placebo-controlled trial. *Lancet* 2005;366:1607-1621.

15. Bhatt DL, Fox KA, Hacke W, et al: Clopidogrel and aspirin versus aspirin alone for the prevention of atherothrombotic events. *N Engl J Med* 2006;354:1706-1717.

16. PRISM-PLUS Study Investigators: Inhibition of the platelet glycoprotein IIb/IIIa receptor with tirofiban in unstable angina and

non-Q-wave myocardial infarction. Platelet Receptor Inhibition in Ischemic Syndrome Management in Patients Limited by Unstable Signs and Symptoms (PRISM-PLUS) study. *N Engl J Med* 1998; 338:1488-1497.

17. PURSUIT Trial Investigators: Inhibition of platelet glycoprotein IIb/IIIa with eptifibatide in patients with acute coronary syndromes. *N Engl J Med* 1998;339:436-443.

18. Roffi M, Chew DP, Mukherjee D, et al: Platelet glycoprotein IIb/IIIa inhibitors reduce mortality in diabetic patients with non-ST-segment-elevation acute coronary syndromes. *Circulation* 2001;104:2767-2771.

19. Bavry AA, Kumbhani DJ, Quiroz R, et al: Invasive therapy along with glycoprotein IIb/IIIa inhibitors and intracoronary stents improves survival in non-ST-segment elevation acute coronary syndromes: a meta-analysis and review of the literature. *Am J Cardiol* 2004;93:830-835.

20. Kendall MJ, Lynch KP, Hjalmarson A, et al: Beta-blockers and sudden cardiac death. *Ann Intern Med* 1995;123:358-367.

21. Beta-Blocker Heart Attack Trial Research Group: A randomized trial of propranolol in patients with acute myocardial infarction. I. Mortality results. *JAMA* 1982;247:1707-1714.

22. Beta-Blocker Heart Attack Trial Research Group: A randomized trial of propranolol in patients with acute myocardial infarction. II. Morbidity results. *JAMA* 1983;250:2814-2819.

23. Gundersen T, Abrahamsen AM, Kjekshus J, et al: Timolol-related reduction in mortality and reinfarction in patients ages 65-75 years surviving acute myocardial infarction. Prepared for the Norwegian Multicentre Study Group. *Circulation* 1982;66:1179-1184.

24. Hjalmarson A, Herlitz J, Holmberg S, et al: The Goteborg metoprolol trial. Effects on mortality and morbidity in acute myocardial infarction. *Circulation* 1983;67:I26-I32.

25. The MIAMI Trial Research Group: Metoprolol in acute myocardial infarction (MIAMI). A randomised placebo-controlled international trial. *Eur Heart J* 1985;6:199-226.

26. Basu S, Senior R, Raval U, et al: Beneficial effects of intravenous and oral carvedilol treatment in acute myocardial infarction. A placebo-controlled, randomized trial. *Circulation* 1997;96:183-191.

27. Dargie HJ: Effect of carvedilol on outcome after myocardial infarction in patients with left-ventricular dysfunction: the CAPRICORN randomised trial. *Lancet* 2001;357:1385-1390.

28.   Otterstad JE, Ford I: The effect of carvedilol in patients with impaired left ventricular systolic function following an acute myocardial infarction. How do the treatment effects on total mortality and recurrent myocardial infarction in CAPRICORN compare with previous beta-blocker trials? *Eur J Heart Fail* 2002;4:501-506.

29.   Poole-Wilson PA, Swedberg K, Cleland JG, et al: Comparison of carvedilol and metoprolol on clinical outcomes in patients with chronic heart failure in the Carvedilol Or Metoprolol European Trial (COMET): randomised controlled trial. *Lancet* 2003;362:7-13.

30.   Echt DS, Liebson PR, Mitchell LB, et al: Mortality and morbidity in patients receiving encainide, flecainide, or placebo. The Cardiac Arrhythmia Suppression Trial (CAST). *N Engl J Med* 1991;324:781-788.

31.   Barron H, Viskin S: Dispelling the myths surrounding the use of beta-blockers in patients after myocardial infarction. *Prev Cardiol* 1998;3:13-15.

32.   Chen J, Marciniak TA, Radford MJ, et al: Beta-blocker therapy for secondary prevention of myocardial infarction in elderly diabetic patients. Results from the National Cooperative Cardiovascular Project. *J Am Coll Cardiol* 1999;34:1388-1394.

33.   Moser M: Angiotensin-converting enzyme inhibitors, angiotensin II receptor antagonists and calcium channel blocking agents: a review of potential benefits and possible adverse reactions. *J Am Coll Cardiol* 1997;29:1414-1421.

34.   Indications for ACE inhibitors in the early treatment of acute myocardial infarction: systematic overview of individual data from 100,000 patients in randomized trials. ACE Inhibitor Myocardial Infarction Collaborative Group. *Circulation* 1998;97:2202-2212.

35.   van Gilst WH, Kingma JH, Peels KH, et al: Which patient benefits from early angiotensin-converting enzyme inhibition after myocardial infarction? Results of one-year serial echocardiographic follow-up from the Captopril and Thrombolysis Study (CATS). *J Am Coll Cardiol* 1996;28:114-121.

36.   Pfeffer MA, Braunwald E, Moye LA, et al: Effect of captopril on mortality and morbidity in patients with left ventricular dysfunction after myocardial infarction. Results of the survival and ventricular enlargement trial. The SAVE Investigators. *N Engl J Med* 1992;327:669-677.

37.   Effect of ramipril on mortality and morbidity of survivors of acute myocardial infarction with clinical evidence of heart failure.

The Acute Infarction Ramipril Efficacy (AIRE) Study Investigators. *Lancet* 1993;342:821-828.

38. Torp-Pedersen C, Kober L: Effect of ACE inhibitor trandolapril on life expectancy of patients with reduced left-ventricular function after acute myocardial infarction. TRACE Study Group. Trandolapril Cardiac Evaluation. *Lancet* 1999;354:9-12.

39. Hall AS, Murray GD, Ball SG: Follow-up study of patients randomly allocated ramipril or placebo for heart failure after acute myocardial infarction. AIRE extension (AIREX) Study. Acute Infarction Ramipril Efficacy. *Lancet* 1997;349:1493-1497.

40. Latini R, Maggioni AP, Flather M, et al: ACE inhibitor use in patients with myocardial infarction. Summary of evidence from clinical trials. *Circulation* 1995;92:3132-3137.

41. Domanski MJ, Exner DV, Borkow CB, et al: Effect of angiotensin converting enzyme inhibition on sudden cardiac death in patients following acute myocardial infarction. A meta-analysis of randomized clinical trials. *J Am Coll Cardiol* 1999;33:598-604.

42. Yusuf S, Sleight P, Pogue J, et al: Effects of an angiotensin-converting-enzyme inhibitor, ramipril, on cardiovascular events in high-risk patients. The Heart Outcomes Prevention Evaluation Study Investigators. *N Engl J Med* 2000;342:145-153.

43. O'Keefe JH, Wetzel M, Moe RR, et al: Should an angiotensin-converting enzyme inhibitor be standard therapy for patients with atherosclerotic disease? *J Am Coll Cardiol* 2001;37:1-8.

44. Braunwald E, Domanski MJ, Fowler SE, et al, for the PEACE Trial Investigators: Angiotensin-converting-enzyme inhibition in stable coronary artery disease. *N Engl J Med* 2004;351:2058-2068.

45. Nguyen KN, Aursnes I, Kjekshus J: Interaction between enalapril and aspirin on mortality after acute myocardial infarction: subgroup analysis of the Cooperative New Scandinavian Enalapril Survival Study II (CONSENSUS II). *Am J Cardiol* 1997;79:115-119.

46. Ambrosioni E, Borghi C, Magnani B: The effect of the angiotensin-converting-enzyme inhibitor zofenopril on mortality and morbidity after anterior myocardial infarction. The Survival of Myocardial Infarction Long-Term Evaluation (SMILE) Study Investigators. *N Engl J Med* 1995;332:80-85.

47. Chinese Cardiac Study Collaborative Group: Oral captopril versus placebo among 13,634 patients with suspected acute myo-

cardial infarction: interim report from the Chinese Cardiac Study (CCS-1). *Lancet* 1995;345:686-687.

48. GISSI-3: effects of lisinopril and transdermal glyceryl trinitrate singly and together on 6-week mortality and ventricular function after acute myocardial infarction. Gruppo Italiano per lo Studio della Sopravvivenza nell'infarto Miocardico. *Lancet* 1994; 343:1115-1122.

49. I SIS-4 Collaborative Group: ISIS-4 (Fourth International Study of Infarct Survival): a randomised factorial trial assessing early oral captopril, oral mononitrate, and intravenous magnesium sulphate in 58,050 patients with suspected acute myocardial infarction. *Lancet* 1995;345:669-685.

50. Dickstein K, Kjekshus J: Effects of losartan and captopril on mortality and morbidity in high-risk patients after acute myocardial infarction: the OPTIMAAL randomised trial. Optimal Trial in Myocardial Infarction with Angiotensin II Antagonist Losartan. *Lancet* 2002;360:752-760.

51. McMurray J, Solomon S, Pieper K, et al: The effect of valsartan, captopril, or both on atherosclerotic events after myocardial infarction: an analysis of the Valsartan in Acute Myocardial Infarction Trial (VALIANT). *J Am Coll Cardiol* 2006;47:726-733.

52. Pitt B, Poole-Wilson PA, Segal R, et al: Effect of losartan compared with captopril on mortality in patients with symptomatic heart failure: randomised trial—the Losartan Heart Failure Survival Study (ELITE II). *Lancet* 2000;355:1582-1587.

53. The RESOLVD Investigators: Effects of metoprolol CR in ischemic and dilated cardiomyopathy. The Randomized Evaluation of Strategies for Left Ventricular Dysfunction (RESOLVD) pilot study. *Circulation* 2000;101:378-384.

54. Pitt B, Remme W, Zannad F, et al: Eplerenone, a selective aldosterone blocker, in patients with left ventricular dysfunction after myocardial infarction. *N Engl J Med* 2003;348:1309-1321.

55. Hansen JF: Treatment with verapamil after an acute myocardial infarction. Review of the Danish studies on verapamil in myocardial infarction (DAVIT I and II). *Drugs* 1991;2:43-53.

56.. Gibson RS, Boden WE, Theroux P, et al: Diltiazem and reinfarction in patients with non-Q-wave myocardial infarction. Results of a double-blind, randomized, multicenter trial. *N Engl J Med* 1986;315:423-429.

57.   Gibson RS, Hansen JF, Messerli F, et al: Long-term effects of diltiazem and verapamil on mortality and cardiac events in non-Q-wave acute myocardial infarction without pulmonary congestion: post hoc subset analysis of the multicenter diltiazem postinfarction trial and the second Danish verapamil infarction trial studies. *Am J Cardiol* 2000;86:275-279.

58.   Leitch JW, McElduff P, Dobson A, et al: Outcome with calcium channel antagonists after myocardial infarction: a community-based study. *J Am Coll Cardiol* 1998;31:111-117.

59.   Buxton AE, Lee KL, Fisher JD, et al: A randomized study of the prevention of sudden death in patients with coronary artery disease. Multicenter Unsustained Tachycardia Trial Investigators. *N Engl J Med* 1999;341:1882-1890.

60.   A comparison of antiarrhythmic-drug therapy with implantable defibrillators in patients resuscitated from near-fatal ventricular arrhythmias. The Antiarrhythmics versus Implantable Defibrillators (AVID) Investigators. *N Engl J Med* 1997;337:1576-1583.

61.   Ceremuzynski L, Kleczar E, Krzeminska-Pakula M, et al: Effect of amiodarone on mortality after myocardial infarction: a double-blind, placebo-controlled, pilot study. *J Am Coll Cardiol* 1992;20:1056-1062.

62.   Farrell TG, Bashir Y, Cripps T, et al: Risk stratification for arrhythmic events in postinfarction patients based on heart rate variability, ambulatory electrocardiographic variables and the signal-averaged electrocardiogram. *J Am Coll Cardiol* 1991;18:687-697.

63.   Bailey JJ, Berson AS, Handelsman H, et al: Utility of current risk stratification tests for predicting major arrhythmic events after myocardial infarction. *J Am Coll Cardiol* 2001;38:1902-1911.

64.   Moss AJ, Zareba W, Hall WJ, et al: Prophylactic implantation of a defibrillator in patients with myocardial infarction and reduced ejection fraction. *N Engl J Med* 2002;346:877-883.

65.   Rossouw JE, Anderson GL, Prentice RL, et al: Risks and benefits of estrogen plus progestin in healthy postmenopausal women: principal results from the Women's Health Initiative randomized controlled trial. *JAMA* 2002;288:321-333.

Chapter **8**

Management of Coronary Risk Factors

Epidemiologic and clinical evidence demonstrates a clear association between established risk factors and coronary heart disease (CHD) or other atherosclerotic vascular diseases. These risk factors include dyslipidemia, hypertension, cigarette smoking, diabetes, obesity, and a sedentary lifestyle. Risk factor modification in patients with clinical CHD comprises secondary prevention, in contrast to intervention in patients without clinical CHD, termed primary prevention. As indicated in Figure 8-1, the impact of hypercholesterolemia is amplified in patients with clinical CHD compared to those without CHD.[1] This phenomenon is also true of the other established risk factors and provides an important impetus for intensive risk factor management for secondary prevention.

Emerging risk factors that may affect prognosis include oxidative stress, hyperhomocysteinemia, inflammatory factors, and procoagulant substances. Current evidence suggests their role in CHD, but confirmation by further studies is required. Many of these studies are in progress. The current status of cardiovascular risk factors is summarized in Table 8-1, according to the evidence for: (1) the association of the risk factor with atherosclerotic cardiovascular disease, and (2) reduction of the disease by modification of the risk factor.

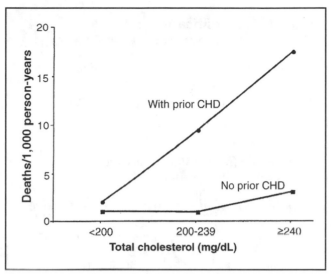

Figure 8-1: Relationship between coronary heart disease (CHD) mortality and total serum cholesterol in populations with and without clinical evidence of prior CHD. From Amsterdam et al, *Am Heart J* 1994;128: 1344-1352, with permission.[1]

Lipid Modification

A large number of clinical trials, primarily with HMG-CoA reductase inhibitors (statins), have convincingly demonstrated that lipid lowering significantly reduces coronary artery disease (CAD) mortality and morbidity in patients with CHD, including those who have had a myocardial infarction (MI). A listing of pertinent clinical trials is presented in Table 8-2.[2]

Pathogenic Mechanisms

Lipid abnormalities play a crucial role in the genesis of atheromatous coronary artery plaques. Hyperlipidemia leads to increased platelet reactivity, endothelial dysfunction, and plaque progression and disruption, all of which

197

Table 8-1: Classification of Cardiovascular Risk Factors

Established–Modification Reduces Clinical Risk
- Cigarette smoking
- Dyslipidemia (elevated LDL cholesterol, low HDL cholesterol)
- Hypertension
- Diabetes (modification reduces risk of microvascular disease)

Probable or Possible–Intervention Data Lacking
- Obesity
- Physical inactivity
- Small, dense LDL cholesterol particles
- Triglycerides
- Homocysteine
- C-reactive protein
- Oxidative stress
- Lipoprotein (a)
- Psychosocial stress
- Infectious agents

Nonmodifiable
- Age
- Sex
- Family history

HDL = high-density lipoprotein
LDL = low-density lipoprotein

facilitate coronary occlusion and acute coronary syndromes (ACS). Oxidized low-density lipoprotein (LDL) particles are a primary factor in these abnormalities, although decreases in high-density lipoprotein (HDL) particles and very-low-density lipoprotein (VLDL) remnants also contribute to atheromatous plaque formation and propagation. The current National Cholesterol Education Program (NCEP) guidelines and update[3,4] recommend a plasma LDL cholesterol (LDL-C) level of <100 mg/dL in patients with atherosclerotic cardiovascular disease. However, endothelial nitric oxide (NO) concentration, necessary for protection against superoxide production, begins to decrease with LDL-C concentrations >40 mg/dL and reaches only approximately 30% of baseline levels at LDL-C concentrations >80 mg/dL. In the presence of oxidized LDL-C, NO concentration decreases sharply to 15% of control levels at LDL-C concentrations >30 mg/dL. Platelet thrombogenic potential is also influenced by LDL-C levels and reversed by statins. Moreover, recent clinical trial information suggests that LDL-C should be substantially lower than that value in patients after acute myocardial infarction (AMI) and other very high risk conditions, specifically <70 mg/dL. For example, as a result of MIRACL[5] and PROVE-IT,[6] post-AMI trials, it has been recommended that even if the LDL-C value initially was <100 mg/dL, it should be lowered by 30% from baseline at time of AMI. Hypercholesterolemia is associated with an increase in thromboxane A_2, a potent platelet activator. Statins reduce thrombus formation in an ex vivo model, largely through antiplatelet activity. Other beneficial effects of statins include a reduction of smooth muscle cell plasminogen activator inhibitor-1 (PAI-1) antigen and an increase in endothelial cell-derived tissue plasminogen activator (tPA), both of which improve thrombolytic balance and may be partially independent of lipid concentration effects.

Table 8-2: Overview of Clinical Trials of Lipid Lowering vs Placebo After Myocardial Infarction

Trial	Subjects	MI (mo)*
POSCH** (1990)[58]	838	6-60
4S† (1994)[10]	4,444	>6
CARE** (1995)[11]	4,159	3-20
LIPID† (1998)[12]	9,014	3-36
VA-HIT† (1999)[59]	2,531	72
L-CAD‡ (2000)[60]	135	6 d
MIRACL† (2001)[5]	2,100	<4 d

POSCH = Program on the Surgical Control of the Hyper-lipidemias: partial intestinal bypass; 4S = Scandinavian Simvastatin Survival Study; CARE = Cholesterol and Recurrent Events; VA-HIT = Veterans Affairs High-Density Lipoprotein Cholesterol Intervention Trial; LIPID = Long-term Intervention with Pravastatin in Ischemic Disease; L-CAD = Lipid-Coronary Artery Disease; MIRACL = Myocardial Ischemia Reduction With Aggressive Cholesterol Lowering; MI = myocardial infarction; RR = relative risk

* = Time from coronary event
** = Outcomes in treatment group vs control group
† = MI or unstable angina
‡ = MI and/or percutaneous transluminal coronary angioplasty secondary to unstable angina

Evidence exists for other vascular effects of statins with the potential for plaque stabilization, such as an increase in endothelial progenitor cells, which could indicate neovascularization of ischemic tissue; a decrease in matrix

Time of Follow-up (y)	Mean/Median Findings**
9.7	[1+2] 35% lower
5.4	[1+2+3] RR 0.66
5	[1+2] 24% lower
6.1	[1] 24% lower
5.1	[1+2] 4% lower
2	[5] 42% lower
16 wk	[1+2+3+4] 16% lower

1 = coronary death; 2 = nonfatal MI; 3 = resuscitated cardiac arrest; 4 = worsening of angina requiring hospitalization; 5 = angiographic progression of coronary atherosclerosis; combined total mortality, cardiovascular death, nonfatal MI, percutaneous coronary intervention/coronary artery bypass grafting, stroke, new onset peripheral vascular disease; [a+b+c] = combined components for outcome data.

From Harjai, *Ann Intern Med* 1999;131:376-386, with permission.[2]

metalloproteinases; and fewer macrophages. Studies of leg blood flow have demonstrated an inverse and continuous relationship between plasma cholesterol level and endothelium-dependent dilatation, with no apparent lower threshold.

Benefits of Lipid Lowering

Meta-analysis of clinical trials has amply demonstrated the efficacy of statins in reducing LDL-C levels. A 10% reduction of serum cholesterol is associated with a 15% reduction in CHD mortality and an 11% reduction in total mortality risk. Several observational studies have also demonstrated the efficacy of early initiation of statin therapy after MI. In the study of the Swedish Registry of Cardiac Intensive Care of almost 20,000 patients, statin treatment initiated by hospital discharge was associated with a mortality of 4.0% (unadjusted) at 1 year compared to 9.3% (unadjusted) in patients discharged without a statin (relative risk reduction, 0.75; P=0.001).[7] Adjusted data indicated a 20% relative reduction in mortality. Lipid measurements were not part of the compulsory data evaluation, but the guidelines for statin intervention were total cholesterol (TC) >200 mg/dL or LDL-C >115 mg/dL. In the Global Use of Strategies to Open Occluded Arteries in Acute Coronary Syndromes (GUSTO IIb) and Platelet Glycoprotein IIb/IIIA in Unstable Angina: Receptor Suppression Using Integrilin Therapy (PURSUIT) trials involving more than 20,000 patients, the odds of dying at 6 months were 33% lower in patients on lipid-lowering agents, with a 20% reduction in the composite outcome of death or nonfatal MI (both results significant).[8] Mortality reduction began at as early as 30 days in the lipid intervention group.

A recently reported trial of lipid lowering in secondary prevention further indicates the general protective effect of lipid lowering. The Heart Protection Study evaluated 20,536 adults with coronary disease, other occlusive arterial disease, or diabetes, randomized to simvastatin (Zocor®) or placebo.[9] After 5 years of follow-up, the statin group demonstrated a reduction in all-cause mortality of 13%, CHD mortality of 18%, nonfatal MI of 27%, and revascularization and stroke of 25%

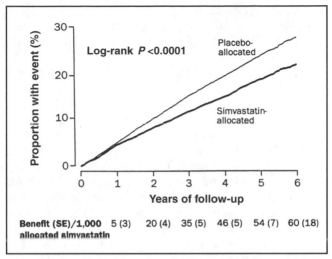

Figure 8-2: Life-table plot of effect of simvastatin allocation on percentages having major vascular events in the Heart Protection Study. From *Lancet* 2002;360:7-22, with permission.[9]

(Figure 8-2). Among the unique and important aspects of this study was confirmation that statin therapy similarly reduced cardiovascular end points in the entire group of patients, regardless of whether initial baseline LDL-C was ≥100 mg/dL or <100 mg/dL. This study provides powerful evidence that lowering LDL-C beyond the current therapeutic target (<100 mg/dL) is beneficial in secondary prevention.

Important post-MI lipid-lowering trials with statins include the Scandinavian Simvastatin Survival Study (4S), the Cholesterol and Recurrent Events (CARE) trial, the Long-term Intervention with Pravastatin in Ischemic Disease (LIPID) study, and the Myocardial Ischemia Reduction with Aggressive Cholesterol Lowering (MIRACL) trial.[5,10-12] The first three trials followed patients with MI or unstable angina (UA), with randomization beginning at least 3 months after the acute event. The MIRACL trial randomized patients within days after the acute event.

All three large, randomized trials demonstrated beneficial effects on primary end points associated with reductions of LDL-C and modest increases in HDL-C. The results of CARE, LIPID, and a primary prevention trial, the West of Scotland Coronary Prevention Study (WOSCOPS), all of which used pravastatin, were pooled to provide enough power to assess specific coronary events.[11-13] This included 19,768 patients and allowed for the evaluation of 2,194 primary end points. Relative risk reduction was similar throughout most of the baseline LDL-C range (125 to 212 mg/dL), with the possible exception of the lowest quintile of the two secondary prevention studies (<125 mg/dL). Relative risk reduction in the treatment group was significantly decreased irrespective of age, gender, smoking history, and diabetes or hypertension status. Pooled analysis of CARE, LIPID, and WOSCOPS demonstrated a reduction of 24% in coronary death and nonfatal infarction vs placebo (95% confidence interval, 14% to 34%; $P=0.005$).[14] There was no significant decrease in event rate for patients with LDL-C <125 mg/dL at baseline.

In contrast with these studies, the MIRACL trial started intensive statin treatment soon after an acute coronary event (24 to 96 hours).[5] A total of 3,086 patients with UA or non-Q-wave MI (53%/54% MI in treatment/placebo groups) who were not candidates for acute coronary revascularization was randomized to high-dose (80 mg) atorvastatin or placebo with evaluation of outcome during the next 16 weeks. The initial LDL-C levels were modestly elevated (124 mg/dL in both groups). The primary combined end point of death, nonfatal MI, cardiac arrest with resuscitation, or recurrent symptomatic myocardial ischemia requiring rehospitalization was 17.4% in the pla-

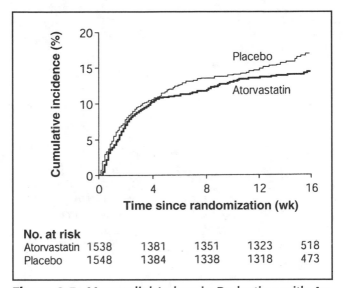

Figure 8-3: Myocardial Ischemia Reduction with Aggressive Cholesterol Lowering (MIRACL) study. Kaplan-Meier estimates of primary outcomes. The relative risk of the composite outcome in the atorvastatin group compared with placebo was 0.84 (95% confidence interval, 0.70 to 1.00; *P*=0.048) based on Cox proportional hazards analysis. The decrease in number at risk at 16 weeks reflects the fact that many patients completed the study within the days immediately preceding 16 weeks. From Schwartz et al, *JAMA* 2001;285: 1711-1718, with permission.[5]

cebo group and 14.8% in the treatment group (*P*=0.048) (Figure 8-3). In terms of individual group outcomes, only the symptomatic ischemia group showed a significant benefit of statin therapy. The changes in lipid levels in the atorvastatin group are of particular interest. The LDL-C values decreased from 124 mg/dL at baseline to 72 mg/dL at the end of the study. Triglycerides fell from 184 mg/dL

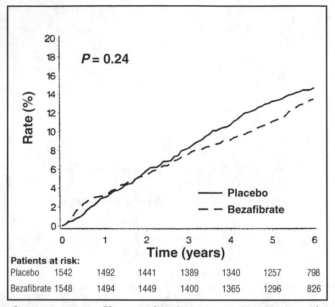

Figure 8-4: Bezafibrate Infarction Prevention (BIP) study. Kaplan-Meier curves for the cumulative probability of the primary event. There was no significant difference. From *Circulation* 2000;102:21-27, with permission.[15]

to 139 mg/dL, and HDL-C increased modestly from 36 mg/dL to 38 mg/dL. The incidence of adverse hepatic effects was 2.5% in the treatment group, which reversed with discontinuation of treatment.

Interestingly, MIRACL demonstrated a significant decrease in stroke in the treatment group (1.6% vs 0.8%), although the incidence was quite low. The high dose of atorvastatin was generally well tolerated, with a serious effect rate of <1% (not significant compared with controls). Although the results did not show a benefit on mortality within this short period, morbidity was significantly reduced. A substantial percentage of patients in each group was on angiotensin-converting enzyme (ACE) inhibitors (49%) and β-blockers (78%), which would tend to minimize the effects of another potential risk-reducing agent. Finally, the largest acceptable dose of the most potent statin was administered and tolerated. It is possible that a similar effect could be achieved with lower doses. This theory is being subjected to further clinical trials.

Evidence from 4S, CARE, and the Air Force/Texas Coronary Atherosclerosis Prevention Study (AFCAPS/TexCAPS) shows significant benefits of risk reduction aimed at decreasing LDL-C, even with low HDL-C levels.[10,11,16] The ratio of TC/HDL-C may be used to guide therapy, in that very-high-risk individuals should have a ratio <4, and high-risk individuals should have a ratio <5. In a study of 3,090 patients with either prior MI (78%) or angina, with triglycerides ≤300 mg/dL, and with low HDL-C (≤45 mg/dL), treatment with bezafibrate or placebo yielded no significant difference in primary end points (fatal MI, nonfatal MI, or sudden death) after 6.2 years, although HDL-C was increased by 19% and triglycerides were reduced by 21%.[15] In the subgroup with triglyceride levels ≥200 mg/dL, however, the reduction in cumulative probability of a primary event with the fibrate was 40% ($P = 0.02$) (Figures 8-4 and 8-5). In the LIPID trial, statins were just as effective in decreasing mortality in patients with high initial triglyceride levels.[12] It is generally recommended that, with LDL-C >130 mg/dL and triglycerides <500 mg/dL, statins are the first choice in secondary prevention, primarily to reduce LDL-C, but also because of their evident beneficial effects on HDL-C and triglycerides. Fibric acids may be reserved as initial therapy for situations in which LDL-C is <100 mg/dL, HDL-C is <40 mg/dL, and triglyceride level is >200 mg/dL, along with aggressive dietary intervention.

Patterns (1998-1999) for use of lipid-lowering medications in patients at hospital discharge after MI were assessed by Fonarow et al.[17] Less than one third of patients received

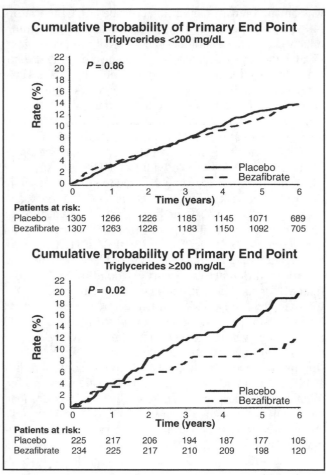

Cumulative Probability of Primary End Point
Triglycerides <200 mg/dL

$P = 0.86$

Patients at risk:

Placebo	1305	1266	1226	1185	1145	1071	689
Bezafibrate	1307	1263	1226	1183	1150	1092	705

Cumulative Probability of Primary End Point
Triglycerides ≥200 mg/dL

$P = 0.02$

Patients at risk:

Placebo	225	217	206	194	187	177	105
Bezafibrate	234	225	217	210	209	198	120

Figure 8-5: Bezafibrate Infarction Prevention (BIP) study. Kaplan-Meier curves for the primary end point in subgroups of patients with baseline triglycerides ≥200 mg/dL and <200 mg/dL. Only in the high baseline triglyceride subgroup were the differences in treatment groups significant. From *Circulation* 2000;102:21-27, with permission.[15]

treatment with these agents. In patients with previous CHD, coronary revascularization, or diabetes, the proportion was higher but still less than 50%. Factors that correlated with the use of lipid-lowering agents included a history of elevated cholesterol, cardiac catheterization during hospitalization, smoking cessation counseling, use of a β-blocker, and care in a teaching hospital.

Recently published relevant clinical trials in AMI or stable CHD have compared either the same statin in different doses or different statins of high and low potency. These trials include PROVE-IT, the A-to-Z trial, the Incremental Decrease in Endpoints through Aggressive Lipid Lowering (IDEAL) trial, and the Treatment to New Targets (TNT) trial.[6,18-20] These trials deal mostly with post-MI patients and involve more than 4,000 to more than 10,000 patients each. They are mostly 5-year follow-up studies evaluating the primary end points of CHD death or nonfatal MI (Table 8-3).

PROVE-IT evaluated 4,162 patients hospitalized for ACS who were randomized to either atorvastatin 80 mg/d or pravastatin 40 mg/d and followed for 18 to 36 months.[6] The median LDL-C level reached during treatment was 95 mg/dL in the pravastatin group, which according to previous standards was acceptable. The atorvastatin group achieved a medial level of 62 mg/dL. A 16% reduction in the primary end point was seen in the atorvastatin group, indicating efficacy of intensive lipid lowering in this patient group.

The A-to-Z trial had a complex protocol involving two phases in patients with ACS.[18] The initial (A) phase involved randomization to enoxaparin or heparin. The second phase, which is relevant here, involved initialization of high-dose (80 mg) or low-dose (20 mg) atorvastatin with follow-up to 24 months. Although a slightly lower percentage of patients experienced the primary end point in the high-simvastatin-dose group, this was not significant over the entire duration of the study, but over the past 20 months the primary end point was significantly reduced in that group.

Table 8-3: Clinical Outcome Trials in Coronary Heart Disease Testing Intensive vs Standard Statin Therapy

Trial	Population	Duration (Y)
PROVE-IT[6]	ACS (4162)	2
A-to-Z[18]	ACS (4497)	2
TNT[21]	SCAD (10,001)	5
IDEAL[20]	SCAD (8888)	5

Comparing both trials, an early benefit was seen in PROVE-IT but not in A-to-Z, but late effect results were similar.[21] The early differences could be explained by the magnitude of C-reactive protein (CRP) lowering (greater difference between groups in PROVE-IT), intensity of early therapy, and differences in early revascularization, rather than by chance.

The IDEAL study evaluated patients with previous MI in Northern Europe who were seen in outpatient facilities.[19] Patients were randomized to atorvastatin 80 mg/d or simvastatin 20 mg/d and followed for a median of 4.8

LDL-C Reduction mg/dL	Risk Reduction in CHD Death or MI (%)
[Potent vs less-potent statin]	
33	16
14	15
24	21
23	11

CHD=coronary heart disease; LDL=low-density lipoprotein cholesterol; MI=myocardial infarction; ACS=acute coronary syndrome; SCAD=stable coronary artery disease. Adapted from Cannon CP: The IDEAL Cholesterol. Lower is better. *JAMA* 2005;294:2492-2494.

years. The major outcome was a major coronary event. Although a slight decrease in the primary end point was seen in the high-dose statin group, it was of borderline significance. However, the high-statin group experienced significantly fewer coronary events in general. The mean levels of LDL-C were 104 mg/dL in the simvastatin group and 81 mg/dL in the atorvastatin group. The results suggested that in patients initiated in aggressive lipid-lowering therapy well beyond the infarct period, although there were no differences in cardiovascular or all-cause mortality, a significant reduction in coronary events in general may ensue without an increase in noncardiovascular mortality or other serious adverse reactions.

The TNT trial evaluated 10,000 patients with CHD, (58% with prior MI), evaluating low-dose atorvastatin (10 mg) vs high-dose (80 mg).[20] A significant reduction in first cardiovascular events developed in the high-dose group. The LDL-C level decreased from a baseline of 152 mg/dL to 101 mg/dL in the low-dose group and to 77 mg/dL in the high dose group. Thus, aggressive management with atorvastatin vs lower dose was effective in decreasing events.

Overall, these studies suggest that more aggressive lowering of LDL-C is beneficial, especially in the acute infarct period. At present, current guidelines suggest that lowering of LDL-C to <70 mg/dL is favored in patients at very high risk— including ACS, established cardiovascular disease with multiple risk factors, especially diabetes, severe and poorly controlled risk factors, and multiple risk factors of the metabolic syndrome.

Several studies in patients with CAD have evaluated the direct effects of high- vs low-potency statins on coronary atheromatous plaques, using serial intravascular ultrasound (IVUS). For example, the REVERSAL (Reversal of Atherosclerosis with Aggressive Lipid Lowering) trial evaluated 502 patients with coronary plaques using randomization to 80 mg atorvastatin or 40 mg pravastatin, the agents and doses also administered in PROVE-IT.[9,22] During 18 months, baseline LDL-C was reduced from 150 mg/dL in the pravastatin group to 110 mg/dl, and to 79 mg/dL in the atorvastatin group. Significantly lower progression rate of coronary atherosclerosis was seen in the high statin group, with the atorvastatin group showing no change in the atheroma burden in comparison with the increase in the pravastatin group. In addition to differences in LDL-C, CRP levels were significantly lower in the atorvastatin group, suggesting a benefit in terms of inflammatory processes.

The most recently developed hydroxymethylglutaryl-coenzyme A (HMG Co-A) reductase inhibitor is rosuvastatin (Crestor®), approved in 2003.[23] Clinical data indicate that it is more potent in lowering LDL-C than any of the other available statins. Pooled results from three trials that included patients with and without CHD and compared rosuvastatin (10 mg) with atorvastatin (10 mg) have been evaluated. As indicated in Figure 8-6, significantly more patients reached their LDL-C goal with rosuvastatin than with atorvastatin (76% vs 53%, P <0.001). Furthermore, the differences in goal achievement were greatest in patients with CAD, in whom the LDL-C goal was <100 mg/dL. In this group, the 10-mg dose of rosuvastatin resulted in achievement of goal in 60% of patients compared to only 19% of patients taking 10 mg of atorvastatin.

The ASTEROID Trial (A Study to Evaluate the Effect of Rosuvastatin on Intravascular Ultrasound-Derived Coronary Atheroma Burden) evaluated 349 patients with coronary lesions treated with intensive statin therapy (rosuvastatin 40 mg/d, with 24-month follow-up).[24] Unlike REVERSAL, no control or comparison drug was used, and the object was evaluation of change in coronary atheroma volume, similar to REVERSAL. LDL-C declined considerably from a baseline of 130 mg/dL to 61 mg/dL. HDL-C levels increased by almost 15%. Significant reductions in percent atheroma volume were found compared with baseline, thus further suggesting that treatment of LDL-C levels to below current guidelines would be beneficial. In fact, the lower levels of LDL-C achieved (61 mg/dL vs 77 mg/dL with atorvastatin in REVERSAL) demonstrated a further benefit in terms of atheroma volume change (Figure 8-7).

Another recent addition to the lipid-lowering armamentarium is ezetimibe (Zetia®). This agent is the first of a new class of drugs that inhibit the intestinal absorption of cholesterol. It is administered in pill form at a dosage of

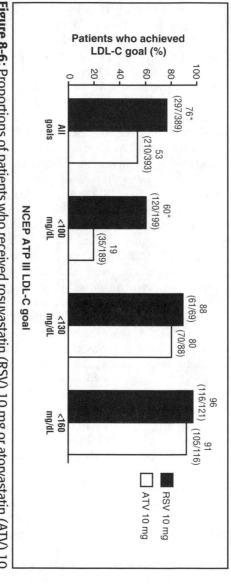

Figure 8-6: Proportions of patients who received rosuvastatin (RSV) 10 mg or atorvastatin (ATV) 10 mg and achieved National Cholesterol Education Program Adult Treatment Panel III (NCEP ATP III) low-density lipoprotein cholesterol (LDL-C) goals at 12 weeks (all goals and by individual goal) based on pooled data from three trials. *P<0.001 vs ATV. Numbers in parentheses are number achieving goal/total number in each category. Mean baseline LDL-C levels were 186 mg/dL for RSV 10 mg and 187 mg/dL for ATV 10 mg. From Shepherd J, Hunninghake DB, Barter P, et al, *Am J Cardiol* 2003;91:11C-17C.[23]

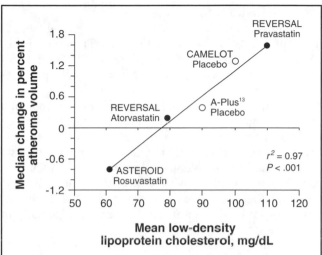

There is a close correlation between these two variables (r^2=0.97). REVERSAL indicates Reversal of Atherosclerosis With Aggressive Lipid-Lowering; CAMELOT=Comparison of Amlodipine vs Enalapril to Limit Occurrences of Thrombosis; A-Plus=Avasimibe and Progression of Lesions on Ultrasound; and ASTEROID=A Study to Evaluate the Effect of Rosuvastatin on Intravascular Ultrasound-Derived Coronary Atheroma Burden.

From Nissen et al: The ASTEROID Trial. *JAMA* 2006;295: 1556-1565.[24]

Figure 8-7: Relationship between mean low-density lipoprotein cholesterol levels and median change in percent atheroma volume for several intravascular ultrasound trials.

10 mg/d. In one study, the administration of ezetimibe with a statin provided an incremental 14% decrease in LDL-C, a 5% increase in HDL-C, and a 10% decrease in triglycerides. Lipid-lowering agents in development include bile acid transport inhibitors and inhibitors of acyl CoA:cholesterol acyltransferase.[25]

Diet and Institutional Issues

Although guidelines for secondary prevention include the implementation of the NCEP Adult Treatment Panel (ATP) III Therapeutic Lifestyle Changes (TLC) diet recommendations[3]—which limit fats to <30% calories, cholesterol to <200 mg, and saturated fats to <7% daily—there is little evidence that this diet is aggressively pursued during hospitalization for MI or after discharge. Issues of nutritional compliance are important. Physicians are generally uncomfortable dealing with nutrition, nutritionists are not usually available in clinical practices, and patient compliance, especially with relatively stringent diets, is low. Nonetheless, there is ample evidence that dietary interventions provide significant risk benefit, especially in secondary prevention.

An example is the Ornish study, involving 48 patients with moderate to severe CAD randomized to intensive lifestyle change vs usual care.[26] The intensive diet consisted of a 10% fat, whole foods, vegetarian diet, aerobic exercise, stress management training, smoking cessation, and group support for 5 years. Coronary arteriograms were evaluated serially. The severity of coronary stenoses decreased in the intensive-treatment group, but increased in the usual-care group. Cardiac events were less common in the intensive-treatment group (risk ratio for control group was 2.5). However, it is highly unlikely that such a regimen could be implemented or followed in an average population compared with this well-motivated volunteer group.

The Mediterranean diet emphasizes more grains, fruit, root and green vegetables, and fish and poultry and less beef, lamb, and pork. Butter is replaced with margarine high in linolenic acid. Based on the results of the Lyon Diet Heart Study, the Lyon diet was important, aside from the results, in specifying the form and types of fat-containing foods and oils.[27] The study evaluated 423 post-MI patients randomized to a Mediterranean-type diet or usual diet. The Lyon diet consisted of 30% fat calories, similar to the American Heart Association (AHA) diet, which is based on the NCEP ATP III recommendations. Saturated fat percentage was also similar (8%), but polyunsaturated fatty acids were lower (<5% vs 7% to 10%), with a cholesterol intake equivalent to the TLC diet (<200 mg). After a mean of 46 months' follow-up, the composite outcome of cardiac stroke and nonfatal MI was reduced (14 events in experimental group, 44 in control group) (Figure 8-8). Major secondary end points, such as stroke, angina, or heart failure, were also significantly reduced in the experimental group. Major traditional risk factors, such as cholesterol levels and hypertension, were independent predictors of outcome events.

The results of the Lyon Diet Heart Study have engendered considerable interest. The key points are:

(1) ω-3 Polyunsaturated fatty acids were important in the beneficial outcomes of this study. The ω-3 fatty acids (fish oils) have demonstrated cardioprotective effects, including decreased dysrhythmias, anti-inflammatory properties, decreased synthesis of cytokines, stimulation of endothelium-derived NO, decreased thrombosis tendency, and inhibition of atherosclerosis.

(2) A 50% to 70% reduction in cardiac end points was noted in the intervention group.

(3) Enhanced definition of the baseline diets of both control and intervention groups is important in analysis. The control group did not have this baseline analysis and was assumed to have a diet equivalent to the treatment group.

(4) Potential geographic and nonmeasured cultural and social differences among treatment populations should be assessed in recommending dietary guidelines. In comparison, the TLC diet, although indicating an increase in polyunsaturated fatty acids, makes no additional recommendation to lower the intake of the ω-6 class of essential fatty acids (linolenic acid), which is high in vegetable oils, nor to increase intake of ω-3 fatty acids (linolenic acid), found in a few vegetable oils such as canola oil, soybean

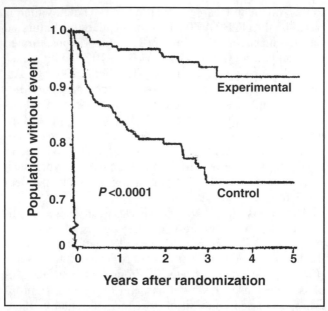

Figure 8-8: Lyon Diet Heart Study. Survival curves for combined cardiac death, nonfatal infarction, unstable angina, heart failure, stroke, and thromboembolism. Log-rank test using the time of the first event was used to compare the control and study (experimental) groups. There was already a striking difference between the two groups within the first year (P<0.0001). From De Lorgeril et al, *J Am Coll Cardiol* 1996;28:1103-1108, with permission.[27]

oil, and flaxseed oil. There is also no comment about the ω-3 fish oils in the TLC diet.

Trans-fatty acids, formed by partial hydrogenation of vegetable oils, have been associated with increased risk for MI. *Trans*-fatty acids constitute 10% to 60% of total fat in margarine and more than 10% of fat in cookies, crackers, French-fried potatoes, glazed doughnuts, and bread. Although investigators agree that *trans*-fatty acids have adverse effects on cholesterol profiles, there is little agreement on the significance of the problem. Food labeling tends to hide the presence of *trans*-fatty acids because they are incorporated under polyunsaturated and monounsaturated fatty acids. *Trans*-fatty acids can be reduced relatively easily by food manufacturers, but substitution of saturated fatty acids should, of course, be avoided.

There is also evidence that the type of protein ingested may beneficially affect cholesterol levels. A meta-analysis of 38 studies on the effects of soy (vegetable) protein intake on serum lipids demonstrated a significant decrease in LDL-C and triglycerides.[28] The effect was strongly related to the initial cholesterol level. It is possible that the beneficial effects on lipids may be the result of isoflavones or phytoestrogens. A recent scientific conference on dietary fatty acids and cardiovascular health provided a concise series of recommendations on this issue. These included efforts by the food industry to genetically modify crops to produce vegetable oils that contain no saturated fat and *trans*-fatty acid-free products. Examples include soybean and canola oils that provide long-chain ω-3 fatty acids. The result could be more heart-healthy products with few essential dietary changes by consumers.

With regard to soy protein, in 1999, the Food and Drug Administration (FDA) approved a health claim that an intake of 25 g/d of soy protein reduces the risk for heart disease.[29]

Stanol/sterol ester-containing foods (called 'nutraceuticals') are emphasized in the NCEP III guidelines for cholesterol management. These components are isolated from soybean oils and esterified to increase solubility. Intakes of 2 to 3 g/d of plant sterols may reduce LDL-C by 10% to 20%, although the effect is inconsistent among individuals. There is little effect on HDL-C or triglycerides. These guidelines recommend that the stanol group be reserved for secondary prevention after an atherosclerotic event.

Recent evaluations of soy protein with isoflavone (phytoestrogen) studies have demonstrated a decrease in LDL-C of about 3%, compared with milk or other proteins, without significant effects on HDL-C, triglycerides, or blood pressure.[29] This was found to be a very small reduction in LDL-C relative to the amount of soy protein evaluated. The conclusion of an AHA science advisory group was that isoflavone supplements in food or pills are not recommended, but that soy products may be beneficial to cardiovascular health because of high content of polyunsaturated fats and fiber and low content of saturated fat.

Antioxidants and Homocysteine Reduction

Considerable interest has been generated about the use of antioxidant vitamins because of evidence that superoxide radicals propagate endothelial damage and lead to atheromatous degeneration and plaque breakdown in the arterial wall. Much of the data on the efficacy of such vitamin supplementation is tenuous. However, a large body of literature has developed on the subject, and it is appropriate to review some highlights in reference to secondary prevention strategies.[29]

The specific vitamins at issue are vitamin E and folic acid. The former has antioxidant properties; the latter decreases homocysteine levels. Because elevated homocysteine levels are a risk factor for coronary events, it seems logical to attempt to lower these levels, which can be accomplished by folic acid, with the support of vitamins B_6 and B_{12}.

Vitamin E (α-Tocopherol)

Several well-designed, epidemiologic studies have demonstrated that high vitamin E consumption is associated with a lower cardiovascular risk. However, randomized, prospective clinical trials have yielded inconsistent results. The Cambridge Heart Antioxidant Study (CHAOS), a randomized, controlled trial of vitamin E in patients with coronary disease, evaluated 2,002 patients with angiographic evidence of CAD to determine the efficacy of high doses of vitamin E in reducing the risk for MI.[30] During approximately 1.5 years, active treatment significantly reduced the risk of cardiovascular death and nonfatal MI (relative risk, 0.53; 95% confidence interval, 0.34 to 0.83). Other studies, notably the Gruppo Italiano per lo Studio della Sopravvivenza nell'Infarto miocardico (GISSI) prevention study, did not demonstrate a significant benefit.[31]

The Heart Protection Study and the Heart Outcomes Prevention Evaluation (HOPE) trial, involving subjects at high risk for coronary events, found no efficacy for vitamin E.[32,33] Moreover, a 3-year trial of 160 patients with CAD and low HDL-C who were randomly assigned to receive antioxidants with lipid-lowering agents demonstrated an attenuation of the protective effect of lipid-lowering therapy when concurrent antioxidants were used (vitamin E, vitamin C, β-carotene, and selenium).[34] In addition, serial coronary angiographic studies indicated that concurrent antioxidants did not significantly attenuate plaque formation, as opposed to the beneficial effect of the lipid-lowering agents alone.[35] An unexpectedly higher all-cause mortality rate was seen in post-menopausal women with coronary disease on hormone replacement therapy given vitamin E and vitamin C compared with women on vitamin placebo.

The HOPE 2 investigators have recently published an extended evaluation of this study to 5 years.[36] There was still no benefit on cardiovascular events even though homocysteine levels were significantly reduced compared with the placebo group.

Folic Acid

Folic acid, vitamin B_6, and vitamin B_{12} serve as cofactors in the enzymatic pathways of homocysteine metabolism. Deficiencies of these cofactors increase homocysteine levels. There is strong evidence that increased homocysteine increases the risk for coronary events and predicts mortality, independent of traditional risk factors in CAD patients (Figure 8-9).[37] There is also evidence for the ben-

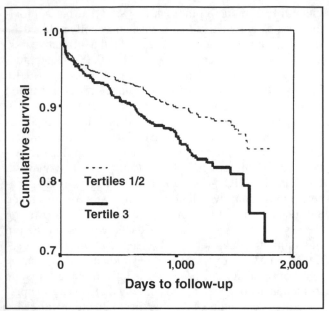

Figure 8-9: Kaplan-Meier survival plots of patients in third homocysteine level (16.2 μg/dL) compared with the first and second tertiles of homocysteine plasma levels from 1,412 patients with severe coronary artery disease. Survival is significantly better in patients in tertiles 1 and 2 (log-rank statistic 10.1, P=0.0014). From Anderson et al, *Circulation* 2000;102:1227-1232, with permission.[37]

eficial effects of folate on coronary atherosclerosis. Although 'normal' homocysteine plasma levels are <15 μmol/L, the primary cardiovascular risk gradient extends below this level. Elevated homocysteine levels have also been associated with increased ischemic myocardial injury in ACS, on the basis of peak cardiac troponin T levels. A recent trial (NORVIT, Norwegian Vitamin Trial of 3,749 men and women given combinations of folic acid, vitamin B_6, vitamin B_{12}, or placebo immediately after AMI with 40-month follow-up) showed no lowering of risk for cardiovascular events after a median follow-up of 40 months, despite significant lowering of homocysteine levels.[38] Moreover, in the group given folic acid, vitamin B_{12}, and vitamin B_6, there was a trend toward an increased relative risk.

Several possible mechanisms for adverse effects of folic acid therapy have included folic acid stimulation of cell proliferation in the atheromatous plaque, effects on methylation potential in vascular cells in mild hyperhomocysteinemic states to promote the development of plaque, and production of asymmetric dimethylarginine, which inhibits NO synthase, thus increasing the risk for vascular disease.[39]

In summary, the results of the use of folic acid and other supplementary B vitamins on cardiovascular risk are disappointing despite lowering of homocysteine levels. It is possible that alternative approaches to decreasing homocysteine levels may provide a more beneficial result.

Hypertension, Diabetes, and Smoking

Hypertension, diabetes, and smoking play major roles in primary and secondary CHD events. The 2001 AHA/American College of Cardiology (ACC) guidelines for secondary prevention are succinct about these three risk factors.[40] The diabetes management goal consists of an HbA_{1c} value <7%, using appropriate hypoglycemic agents and lifestyle modifications to help attain this goal, such as weight management and physical activity. For smoking, the goal is obviously complete cessation using available means, including counseling, nicotine replacement, and bupropion (Zyban®).

Hypertension and Left Ventricular Hypertrophy

The *Seventh Report of the Joint National Committee on Prevention, Detection, Evaluation, and Treatment of High Blood Pressure* provides the following key recommendations for patients with CHD.[41] Blood pressure goal is <140/90 mm Hg. Patients with diabetes or chronic kidney disease should have a target goal of <130/80 mm Hg. The first drugs of choice are usually β-blockers (non-intrinsic sympathomimetic) and angiotensin-converting enzyme (ACE) inhibitors. An aldosterone antagonist and/or a thiazide diuretic is also recommended. Alternatively, long-acting calcium-channel blockers (CCBs) can be used. Short-acting CCBs should be avoided. Nondihydropyridines (verapamil [Calan®, Covera®, Isoptin®, Verelan®] and diltiazem [Cardizem®, Cartia®, Dilacor®, Diltia®, Tiazac®]) have been advocated for hypertension with non-Q-wave MI. The use of calcium-channel antagonists is reviewed in Chapter 7. It should also be noted that the ACC/AHA 2002 guidelines for management of UA and non-ST-segment elevation MI recommend a general target blood pressure of <135/85 mm Hg for all patients with ACS.[42]

Whether lowering blood pressure well below 140/90 mm Hg would be beneficial in patients after MI is not known. The Hypertension Optimal Treatment (HOT) study, in which 8% of patients had CHD and <2% had previous MI, demonstrated no adverse effects and, in fact, a decrease in adverse cardiac events when diastolic blood pressure had decreased to a mean of 83 mm Hg.[43] However, the small percentage of patients with prior MI in this group precludes extrapolation of the results to MI patients in general.

An intriguing study (CAMELOT, Comparison of amlodipine vs enalapril to limit occurrences of thrombosis) in 1,991 patients with stable CAD and normal blood pressures randomized patients to the CCB amlodipine 10 mg/d, or the ACE inhibitor enalapril 20 mg/d. Baseline blood pressure was 129/78 mm Hg in both groups.[44] The results suggested benefit for the CCB because of a significant decrease in cardiovascular events in the CCB group (hazard ratio 0.69, 95% CI 0.54-0.88). Additionally, an IVUS substudy showed a trend toward less progression of atherosclerosis in the amlodipine group, and a borderline progression in the enalapril group. The results of CAMELOT and PEACE[45] raise some question about the recommendation for ACE inhibitors in stable CAD patients, especially if robust use of other cardioprotective agents is initiated or continued.

Another concern is the effect of left ventricular hypertrophy (LVH) on prognosis. A substantial proportion of patients with hypertension (20% to 30%) have echocardiographic evidence for LVH. LVH is a significant, independent risk factor for adverse cardiac events regardless of whether a patient has had an MI. Although LVH appears to affect women more profoundly than men in the absence of CAD, there is no definitive information on the gender-related impact of differences in LVH in MI patients. It has been demonstrated that hypertension with LVH is associated with coronary vascular remodeling and attenuated endothelial and nonendothelial coronary flow reserve.

Based on these considerations, we recommend the initial use of β-blockers as antihypertensive agents after MI, with appropriate conjunctive use of ACE inhibitors. If either of these classes is contraindicated, we would administer long-acting CCBs instead of β-blockers. Whether to use a dihydropyridine or a nondihydropyridine should be determined by factors such as the patient's baseline heart rate. Angiotensin II receptor blockers (ARBs) could be substituted for ACE inhibitors if side effect issues arise. If there is additional evidence for congestive heart failure (CHF) or poor left ventricular ejection fraction (LVEF) and the blood pressure remains elevated, efforts should be made to carefully optimize blood pressure levels to <130/85 to decrease myocardial oxygen needs by decreasing afterload. Thiazide diuretics are usually more effective than loop diuretics in reducing blood pressure, but, if creatinine levels are >2.0 or if significant CHF is present, a loop diuretic would be a better choice. Of course, salt restriction to <6 g/d is important in hypertension, regardless of whether CHF is present.

Diabetes

Type 2 diabetes, which accounts for 85% of diabetes cases, is an important risk factor for CHD, stroke, and peripheral vascular disease. The occurrence of MI in patients with diabetes is often associated with subtle symptoms, frequently with little evidence of chest discomfort. According to current NCEP guidelines, patients with diabetes and without prior CHD are now considered to be CHD 'equivalents' with identical risk reduction targets. The evidence for this approach is the equal incidence rates of MI in subjects without diabetes and with previous MI and in patients with diabetes and without previous MI.[46] In a study of 4,000 MI patients in Finland (15% with diabetes), it was found that the 28-day mortality was 14% in diabetic men and 9% in nondiabetic men.[47] In diabetic and nondiabetic women, mortality was 22% and 8%, respectively. In one half of patients with diabetes who die within 1 year of a first cardiac event, death is sudden. With the rising prevalence of diabetes in the United States, these findings have assumed an increasing importance.

In treating type 2 diabetes, the physician must deal with insulin deficiency and insulin resistance. Insulin resistance leads to increased insulin levels, which could have adverse effects on blood pressure and the endothelium, as well as on lipid levels. Insulin resistance can be reduced by weight reduction, when appropriate, and exercise.

Hyperglycemia is controlled by insulin and several groups of oral hypoglycemic agents, including the α-glucosidases and thiazolidinediones (TZDs). The former reduce glucose absorption, and the latter increase tissue sensitivity to insulin. Metformin (Glucophage®), a biguanide, has been useful in decreasing microvascular disease events in overweight patients with diabetes. The sulfonylureas increase pancreatic β-cell insulin release.

In the MICRO-HOPE trial, patients with diabetes and at least one other risk factor for cardiovascular disease who were treated with the ACE inhibitor ramipril (Altace®) had a significant reduction in cardiovascular death (37%), nonfatal MI (22%), stroke (33%), and total mortality (24%) compared with a placebo group during 4.5 years.[48] The use of ACE inhibitors also appears to decrease the development of albuminuria and overt nephropathy, as well as the development of diabetes, based on analysis of the HOPE study. Moreover, patients with diabetes treated with ACE inhibitors within 24 hours of MI in the GISSI-3 trial had a reduced 6-week mortality (8.7% vs 12.4% treated conventionally).[49]

Based on these considerations, it is recommended that the post-MI patient with diabetes receive aggressive control of blood sugar, with HbA_{1c} levels maintained at <7%. Metformin, among other agents, appears to have properties for risk reduction and should be used if there is no contraindication. High-fiber foods and foods with a low glycemic index should be emphasized, based on changes in blood sugar 3 hours after consumption of a reference food containing 50 g of available carbohydrate. The use of ACE inhibitors, beginning in the hospital, is also strongly recommended.

Smoking

Health-care personnel recognize how difficult smoking cessation is for patients, although post-MI patients are more likely to stop than those with CHD who have not developed an ACS. However, smoking is the leading preventable cause of CAD and death in the industrialized world. There is compelling evidence that, in addition to adverse effects on platelet function and production of carboxyhemoglobin, the inhaled products of smoking, specifically nicotine, cause acute endothelial dysfunction. Cigarette smoking in general causes epicardial coronary artery constriction by stimulating coronary β-adrenergic receptors. Oxidative stress may mediate the effects on endothelial dysfunction caused by smoking, possibly associated with NO synthase inhibition.

Because there is no argument about the necessity of smoking cessation, especially after an MI, the challenge is how to achieve success. Perhaps the most comprehensive analysis of successful cessation interventions was accomplished by Kottke et al in 1988.[50] They used a meta-analysis of 108 intervention comparisons in 39 controlled smoking cessation trials. The best results were achieved by multiple intervention techniques involving a team of physicians and nonphysicians. A combination of group and individual sessions had the greatest chance of success at 12 months. These trials used nicotine chewing gum extensively, but the nicotine patch was not yet widely used. The meta-analysis found that, at 12 months, the average difference in quit rate between intervention and control groups was just under 6%, although there was considerable variation in individual programs, with the greatest difference being 50%. Reinforcement and frequent contacts appear to increase successful compliance.

A study of a nurse-managed program concluded that such a program after MI was highly cost-effective in terms of lives saved, even if the program decreased the smoking rate by only 3/1,000 smokers (assuming a baseline of 26% smokers).[51]

Considering the increasing encroachment on a physician's time by administrative duties and other responsibilities, it seems reasonable to try to develop comprehensive smoking cessation programs early in the post-MI period and, perhaps, to extend the efforts through hospital-based contact after the patient has been discharged.

The best approach that an individual physician can take in dealing with a patient who persists in smoking is to: (1) provide a quit-smoking message with each patient contact, (2) attempt to set a quit-smoking date if the patient agrees, (3) reinforce this decision by telephone contact, and (4) provide group and individual health-professional

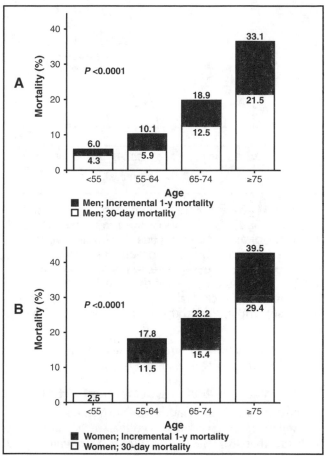

Figure 8-10: Sex differences in mortality after acute myocardial infarction in 2,867 consecutive patients from the Israeli Thrombolytic Survey Group Study. Thirty-day and 1-year crude mortality rates by age subgroups in (A) men and (B) women. *P* for trend <0.0001 for 30-day mortality and incremental 1-year mortality rates in both sexes. From Gottlieb et al, *Circulation* 2000;102:2484-2490, with permission.[52]

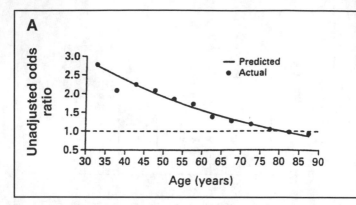

Figure 8-11: National Registry of Myocardial Infarction 2 (1994-1998). Odds ratio (women:men) for death during hospitalization for myocardial infarction, according to age. Risk ratio for women compared to men increased with decreasing age, reaching >2 at <35 years old. The unadjusted odds ratios (A) were derived from the model that included sex, age, the interaction between sex and age, and the year of discharge. The ad-

support through the following year, with the assistance of nicotine patches and bupropion if needed.

Gender Issues in Acute Myocardial Infarction

Substantial evidence indicates that women with acute MI are less aggressively managed than men. Information from the charts of 138,956 Medicare beneficiaries with AMI in 1994 and 1995 indicated a decreased likelihood of interventional procedures in women of all age groups.[53] Many of these differences were small, however, and early mortality was not affected. Further studies indicate that, in female MI patients who are older, have a greater prevalence of risk factors, and have a higher complication rate, there is no difference in aspirin use, β-blocker administration, or interventional procedures. In the Israeli Throm-

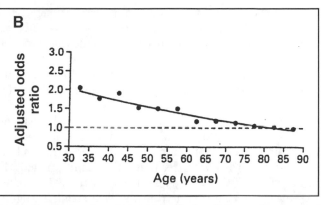

B

justed odds ratios (B) were derived from the model that included race, insurance status, medical history, severity of clinical abnormalities at admission, type of management in the first 24 hours after admission, and time of presentation. As seen in B, the adjusted odds ratios indicated a greater relative risk of mortality in women up to age 80. From Vaccarino et al, *N Engl J Med* 1999;341:217-225, with permission.[55]

bolytic Survey Group Study, the 30-day mortality, but not the 1-year mortality, was higher for women (Figure 8-10).[52] The difference in early outcome was explained by the older age of the women and greater comorbidity. There is also evidence that women with angina are less likely to undergo diagnostic cardiac catheterization. This is especially salient because women experience chest pain as a symptom of CAD more commonly than men. One possible explanation for the discrepancy in diagnostic catheterization is the greater likelihood of normal epicardial coronary arteries in women with chest pain. Finally, stress test specificities tend to be lower in women than men (more false-positive tests). In terms of response to acute interventions, there have been concerns about a higher incidence of coronary reocclusion or complications after post-MI interventions. However, an evaluation of coronary patency rates of the infarct-related artery after thrombolysis indicated no significant gender difference at 90 minutes and at 5 to 7 days after the intervention.

Although women are less likely to have MI as the initial presentation of CAD, they have a higher fatality rate. Whether this is due to more atypical presentations in women or to the lower likelihood of women to seek medical attention for these symptoms is unclear. Biennial evaluation of the Framingham population, allowing for retrospective evaluation of MI incidence, found that unrecognized MI occurred in 38% of women compared with 28% of men. However, a recent report from the Heart and Estrogen/Progestin Replacement Study (HERS) of 2,763 postmenopausal women with CAD found that only 4.3% of women with nonfatal MI were unrecognized, based on serial electrocardiograms (ECG) and hospitalization information.[54]

An analysis of 384,878 patients enrolled in the US National Registry of Myocardial Infarction 2 between 1994 and 1998 showed a higher mortality in hospitalized women than in men (16.7% vs 11.5%).[55] Younger women (<50 years) were more likely to die in the hospital than men of similar age (Figure 8-11). This difference decreased with age, and mortality rates were similar after age 74. After accounting for differences in medical history, severity of the MI, and management, risk was still higher in younger women. Indeed, after adjustment for these factors, one third of the risk difference was still unexplained. Possible reasons for the higher in-hospital mortality for younger women may relate to the underlying pathophysiologic state, including clotting mechanisms and the type of plaque disruption.

In an analysis of 6,826 patients discharged after MI, 2-year mortality was higher in women than in men (29% vs 20%).[56] As with the hospitalization period in other studies, only younger women had a higher posthospitalization mortality than men of similar age, with the sex difference in mortality decreasing with increasing age. This relationship held after adjustment for demographic characteristics and medical history. Unfortunately, there was no information on smoking patterns after hospitalization or posthospital treatment and compliance, which could have affected outcomes.[57]

Diagnosis of ischemic heart disease remains a challenge because of gender differences in reporting of chest pain, which is less likely to be associated with flow-limiting coronary stenosis in women.[57] However the Women's Ischemic Syndrome Evaluation (WISE) study and other evaluations have suggested the presence of endothelial dysfunction and impaired coronary flow reserve with chest pain with no evidence of flow-limiting stenosis. The increased emphasis on differences in presentation of ischemic symptoms, prognosis after AMI, and intervention in women and men should lead to more effective diagnostic and treatment strategies in women.

References

1. Amsterdam EA, Hyson D, Kappagoda CT: Nonpharmacologic therapy for coronary artery atherosclerosis: results of primary and secondary prevention trials. *Am Heart J* 1994;128:1344-1352.

2. Harjai KJ: Potential new cardiovascular risk factors: left ventricular hypertrophy, homocysteine, lipoprotein(a), triglycerides, oxidative stress, and fibrinogen. *Ann Intern Med* 1999;131:376-386.

3. National Cholesterol Education Program (NCEP) Expert Panel on Detection, Evaluation, and Treatment of High Blood Cholesterol in Adults (Adult Treatment Panel III). Third Report of the National Cholesterol Education Program (NCEP) Expert Panel on Detection, Evaluation, and Treatment of High Blood Cholesterol in Adults (Adult Treatment Panel III) final report. http://www.nhlbi.nih.gov/guidelines/cholesterol/atp3_rpt.htm. Accessed September 9, 2006.

4. Grundy SM, Cleeman JI, Merz CN, et al: Implications of recent clinical trials for the National Cholesterol Education Program Adult Treatment Panel III guidelines. *Circulation* 2004;110:227-239. [Published correction appears in *Circulation* 2004; 110:763].

5. Schwartz GG, Olsson AG, Ezekowitz MD, et al: Effects of atorvastatin on early recurrent ischemic events in acute coronary

syndromes: the MIRACL study: a randomized controlled trial. *JAMA* 2001;285:1711-1718.

6. Cannon CP, Braunwald E, McCabe CH, et al, for the Pravastatin or Atorvastatin Evaluation and infection Therapy-Thrombolysis in Myocardial Infarction 22 investigators: Intensive versus moderate lipid lowering with statins after acute coronary syndromes. *N Engl J Med* 2004;350:1495-1504.

7. Stenestrand U, Wallentin L: Early revascularisation and 1-year survival in 14-day survivors of acute myocardial infarction: a prospective cohort study. *Lancet* 2002;359:1805-1811.

8. Aronow HD, Topol EJ, Roe MT, et al: Effect of lipid-lowering therapy on early mortality after acute coronary syndromes: an observational study. *Lancet* 2001;357:1063-1068.

9. Heart Protection Study Collaborative Group: MRC/BHF Heart Protection Study of cholesterol lowering with simvastatin in 20,536 high-risk individuals—a randomised placebo-controlled trial. *Lancet* 2002;360:7-22.

10. Randomised trial of cholesterol lowering in 4444 patients with coronary heart disease: the Scandinavian Simvastatin Survival Study (4S). *Lancet* 1994;344:1383-1389.

11. Sacks FM, Pfeffer MA, Moye LA, et al: The effect of pravastatin on coronary events after myocardial infarction in patients with average cholesterol levels. Cholesterol and Recurrent Events Trial investigators. *N Engl J Med* 1996;335:1001-1009.

12. Prevention of cardiovascular events and death with pravastatin in patients with coronary heart disease and a broad range of initial cholesterol levels. The Long-Term Intervention with Pravastatin in Ischaemic Disease (LIPID) Study Group. *N Engl J Med* 1998;339:1349-1357.

13. WOSCOPS Group: Influence of pravastatin and plasma lipids on clinical events in the West of Scotland Coronary Prevention Study (WOSCOPS). *Circulation* 1998;97:1440-1445.

14. Simes J, Furberg CD, Braunwald E: Effects of pravastatin on mortality in patients with and without coronary heart disease across a broad range of cholesterol levels. The Prospective Pravastatin Pooling Project. *Eur Heart J* 2002;23:207-215.

15. Secondary prevention by raising HDL cholesterol and reducing triglycerides in patients with coronary artery disease: the Bezafibrate Infarction Prevention (BIP) study. *Circulation* 2000;102:21-27.

16. Downs JR, Clearfield M, Weis S, et al: Primary prevention of acute coronary events with lovastatin in men and women with average cholesterol levels: results of Air Force/Texas Coronary Atherosclerosis Prevention Study (AFCAPS/TexCAPS). *JAMA* 1998;279:1615-1622.

17. Fonarow GC, French WJ, Parsons LS, et al: Use of lipid-lowering medications at discharge in patients with acute myocardial infarction: data from the National Registry of Myocardial Infarction 3. *Circulation* 2001;103:38-44.

18. de Lemos JA, Blazing MA, Wiviott SD, et al: Early intensive versus delayed conservative simvastatin strategy in patients with acute coronary syndromes: phase Z of the A to Z trial. *JAMA* 2004;292:1307-1316.

19. Pedersen TR, Faergeman O, Kastelein JJ, et al: High-dose atorvastatin vs usual- dose simvastatin for secondary prevention after myocardial infarction: the IDEAL study: a randomized controlled trial. *JAMA* 2005;294:2437-2445.

20. LaRosa JC, Grundy SM, Waters DD, et al: Intensive lipid lowering with atorvastatin in patients with stable coronary disease. *N Engl J Med* 2005;352:1425-1435.

21. Wiviott SD, de Lemos JA, Cannon CP, et al: A tale of two trials: a comparison of the post-acute coronary syndrome lipid-lowering trials A to Z and PROVE IT-TIMI 22. *Circulation* 2006; 113:1406-1414.

22. Nissen SE, Tuzcu EM, Schoenhagen P, et al for the REVERSAL investigators: Effect of intensive compared with moderate lipid-lowering therapy on progression of coronary atherosclerosis. A randomized controlled trial. *JAMA* 2004;291:1071-1080.

23. Shepherd J, Hunninghake DB, Barter P, et al: Guidelines for lowering lipids to reduce coronary artery disease risk: a comparison of rosuvastatin with atorvastatin, pravastatin, and simvastatin for achieving lipid-lowering goals. *Am J Cardiol* 2003;91:11C-17C.

24. Nissen SE, Nicholls SJ, Sipahi I, et al: For the ASTEROID investigators. Effect of very high-intensity statin therapy on regression of coronary atherosclerosis. The ASTEROID trial. *JAMA* 2006;295:1556-1565.

25. Kerzner B, Corbelli J, Sharp S, et al: Efficacy and safety of ezetimibe coadministered with lovastatin in primary hypercholesterolemia. *Am J Cardiol* 2003;91:418-424.

26. Ornish D, Scherwitz LW, Billings JH, et al: Intensive lifestyle changes for reversal of coronary heart disease. *JAMA* 1998;280: 2001-2007.

27. De Lorgeril M, Salen P, Martin JL, et al: Effect of a Mediterranean type of diet on the rate of cardiovascular complications in patients with coronary artery disease. Insights into the cardioprotective effect of certain nutriments. *J Am Coll Cardiol* 1996;28:1103-1108.

28. Sacks FM, Lichtenstein A, Van Horn L, et al, for the American Heart Association Nutrition Committee: Soy protein, isoflavones, and cardiovascular health. An American Heart Association science advisory for professionals from the Nutrition Committee. *Circulation* 2006;113:1034-1044.

29. Kris-Etherton PM, Lichtenstein AH, Howard BV, et al: Antioxidant vitamin supplements and cardiovascular disease. *Circulation* 2004;110:637-641.

30. Stephens NG, Parsons A, Schofield PM, et al: Randomised controlled trial of vitamin E in patients with coronary disease. Cambridge Heart Antioxidant Study (CHAOS). *Lancet* 1996;347: 781-786.

31. Gruppo Italiano per lo Studio della Sopravvivenza nell'Infarto miocardico: Dietary supplementation with n-3 polyunsaturated fatty acids and vitamin E after myocardial infarction—results of the GISSI-Prevenzione trial. *Lancet* 1999;354:447-455. [Published erratum in *Lancet* 2001;357:642.]

32. MRC/BHF Heart Protection Study: Antioxidant vitamin supplementation in 20,536 high-risk individuals—a randomised placebo-controlled trial. *Lancet* 2002;360:23-33.

33. Yusuf S, Dagenais G, Pogue J, et al: Vitamin E supplementation and cardiovascular events in high-risk patients. Heart Outcomes Prevention Evaluation (HOPE) Study Investigators. *N Engl J Med* 2000;342:154-160.

34. Brown BG, Zhao XQ, Chait A, et al: Simvastatin and niacin, antioxidant vitamins, or the combination for the prevention of coronary disease. *N Engl J Med* 2001;345:1583-1592.

35. Waters DD, Alderman EL, Hsia J, et al: Effects of hormone replacement therapy and antioxidant vitamin supplements on coronary atherosclerosis in postmenopausal women—a randomized controlled trial. *JAMA* 2002;288:2432-2440.

36.   Lonn E, Yusuf S, Arnold MJ, et al: Homocysteine lowering with folic acid and B vitamins in vascular disease. Heart Outcomes Prevention Evaluation (HOPE) 2 Study Investigators. *New Engl J Med* 2006;354:1567-1577.

37.   Anderson JL, Muhlestein JB, Horne BD, et al: Plasma homocysteine predicts mortality independently of traditional risk factors and C-reactive protein in patients with angiographically defined coronary artery disease. *Circulation* 2000;102:1227-1232.

38.   Bønaa KH, Njølstad I, Ueland PM, et al for the NORVIT trial investigators: Homocysteine lowering and cardiovascular events after myocardial infarction. *N Eng J Med* 2006;354:1578-1588.

39.   Loscalzo J: Homocysteine trials—clear outcomes for complex reasons. *N Engl J Med* 2006;354:1629-1632.

40.   Smith SC Jr, Blair SN, Bonow RO, et al: AHA/ACC Guidelines for Preventing Heart Attack and Death in Patients With Atherosclerotic Cardiovascular Disease: 2001 update. A statement for healthcare professionals from the American Heart Association and the American College of Cardiology. *J Am Coll Cardiol* 2001;38:1581-1583.

41.   Chobanian AV, Bakris GL, Black HR, et al: The Seventh Report of the Joint National Committee on Prevention, Detection, Evaluation, and Treatment of High Blood Pressure. *JAMA* 2003;289:2560-2572.

42.   Braunwald E, Antman EM, Beasley JW, et al: ACC/AHA 2002 guideline update for the management of patients with unstable angina and non-ST-segment elevation myocardial infarction: a report of the American College of Cardiology/American Heart Association Task Force on Practice Guidelines (Committee on the Management of Patients With Unstable Angina). *J Am Coll Cardiol* 2002;40:1366-1374.

43.   Hansson L, Zanchetti A, Carruthers SG, et al: Effects of intensive blood-pressure lowering and low-dose aspirin in patients with hypertension: principal results of the Hypertension Optimal Treatment (HOT) randomised trial. HOT Study Group. *Lancet* 1998;351:1755-1762.

44.   Nissen SE, Tuzcu EM, Libby P, et al: CAMELOT investigators. Effect of antihypertensive agents on cardiovascular events in patients with coronary disease and normal blood pressure: the CAMELOT study: a randomized controlled trial. *JAMA* 2004;292:2217-2225.

45. Braunwald E, Domanski MJ, Fowler SE, et al: Angiotensin-converting-enzyme inhibition in stable coronary artery disease. PEACE Trial Investigators. *N Engl J Med* 2004;351:2058-2068.

46. Haffner SM, Lehto S, Ronnemaa T, et al: Mortality from coronary heart disease in subjects with type 2 diabetes and in nondiabetic subjects with and without prior myocardial infarction. *New Engl J Med* 1998;339:229-234.

47. Miettinen H, Lehto S, Salomaa V, et al: Impact of diabetes on mortality after the first myocardial infarction. FINMONICA Myocardial Infarction Register Study Group. *Diabetes Care* 1998;21:69-75.

48. Effects of ramipril on cardiovascular and microvascular outcomes in people with diabetes mellitus: results of the HOPE study and MICRO-HOPE substudy. Heart Outcomes Prevention Evaluation (HOPE) Study Investigators. *Lancet* 2000;355:253-259. [Erratum in *Lancet* 2000;356:860].

49. Zuanetti G, Latini R, Maggioni AP, et al: Effect of the ACE inhibitor lisinopril on mortality in diabetic patients with acute myocardial infarction—data from the GISSI-3 study. *Circulation* 1997;96:4239-4245.

50. Kottke TE, Battista RN, DeFriese GH, et al: Attributes of successful smoking cessation interventions in medical practice. A meta-analysis of 39 controlled trials. *JAMA* 1988;259:2883-2889.

51. Taylor CB, Houston-Miller N, Killen JD, et al: Smoking cessation after acute myocardial infarction—effects of a nurse-managed intervention. *Ann Intern Med* 1990;113:118-123.

52. Gottlieb S, Harpaz D, Shotan A, et al: Sex differences in management and outcome after acute myocardial infarction in the 1990s: A prospective observational community-based study. Israeli Thrombolytic Survey Group. *Circulation* 2000;102:2484-2490.

53. Gan SC, Beaver SK, Houck PM, et al: Treatment of acute myocardial infarction and 30-day mortality among women and men. *N Engl J Med* 2000;343:8-15.

54. Hulley S, Grady D, Bush T, et al: Randomized trial of estrogen plus progestin for secondary prevention of coronary heart disease in postmenopausal women. Heart and Estrogen/progestin Replacement Study (HERS) Research Group. *JAMA* 1998;280:605-613.

55. Vaccarino V, Parsons L, Every NR, et al: Sex-based differences in early mortality after myocardial infarction. National Reg-

istry of Myocardial Infarction 2 Participants. *N Engl J Med* 1999;341:217-225.

56. Vaccarino V, Krumholz HM, Yarzebski J, et al: Sex differences in 2-year mortality after hospital discharge for myocardial infarction. *Ann Intern Med* 2001;134:173-181.

57. Bairey Merz NB, Bonow RO, Sopko G, et al: Women's Ischemic Syndrome Evaluation: current status and future research directions: report from the National Heart, Lung and Blood Institute workshop. *Circulation* 2004;109:805-807.

58. Buchwald H, Varco RL, Matts JP, et al: Effect of partial ileal bypass surgery on mortality and morbidity from coronary heart disease in patients with hypercholesterolemia. Report of the Program on the Surgical Control of the Hyperlipidemias (POSCH). *N Engl J Med* 1990;323:946-955.

59. Rubins HB, Robins SJ, Collins D, et al: Gemfibrozil for the secondary prevention of coronary heart disease in men with low levels of high-density lipoprotein cholesterol. Veterans Affairs High-Density Lipoprotein Cholesterol Intervention Trial Study Group. *N Engl J Med* 1999;341:410-418.

60. Arntz HR, Agrawal R, Wunderlich W, et al: Beneficial effects of pravastatin (+/-colestyramine/niacin) initiated immediately after a coronary event. The Randomized Lipid-Coronary Artery Disease (L-CAD) Study. *Am J Cardiol* 2000;86:1293-1298.

Chapter **9**

Risks and Pathophysiology of Heart Failure

Despite our ability to recognize the presence of heart failure by a constellation of typical signs and symptoms, the definitions used to describe this syndrome have evolved substantially over time. This redefinition of heart failure is based on observations made by astute clinicians and on results of clinical trials assessing new therapies. Recently, our understanding of the basis of heart failure has been extended by insights gained using the techniques of molecular biology and by pioneering work defining the human genome.

The continued evolution of our understanding of heart failure pathophysiology has resulted in a succession of paradigms to describe this syndrome. Figure 9-1 depicts the paradigms that have been used over the past 50 years. These paradigms help us clinically because they provide a rationale for many of the therapies that are now being used or evaluated for the treatment of heart failure. However, in reality, no single paradigm suffices as a complete description of heart failure. All are correct, but none are by themselves sufficient. Thus, depending on the purpose, a clinician might use one or more of these paradigms to help explain a particular clinical or mechanistic aspect of heart failure. As we shall see, however, the neurohormonal model of heart failure that has been developed over the past 20 years dominates our thinking about heart failure

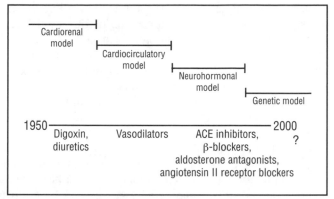

Figure 9-1: Heart failure paradigms.

pathophysiology and has provided a basis for many of the new and highly effective therapies that have emerged for its treatment.

A useful definition proposed by Philip Poole-Wilson in 1985 defined heart failure as "a clinical syndrome caused by an abnormality of the heart and recognized by a characteristic pattern of haemodynamic, renal, neural, and hormonal responses." This definition incorporates many aspects of the cardiorenal, cardiocirculatory, and neurohormonal paradigms depicted in Figure 9-1 and could be further extended by adding that when heart failure develops, the heart is unable to provide adequate amounts of oxygenated blood to meet the needs of peripheral tissue or is able to do so only at abnormally high intracardiac filling pressures.

It is worth pointing out that the term *heart failure* rather than *congestive heart failure* is used in this definition and throughout the remaining chapters of this handbook because many patients with heart failure may not have evidence of congestion. For example, a patient with acutely decompensated heart failure caused by severely depressed left ventricular systolic function (LVSF) is admitted to the hospital with pulmonary edema and is subsequently diuresed so that signs and symptoms of volume overload are abolished. In this case, many of the abnormalities in cardiac structure and function, circulatory hemodynamics, and neurohormonal activation persist despite the resolution of congestive signs and symptoms. The issue is more than merely a semantic one, because many physicians might be tempted to consider this patient to be free of heart failure (and at low risk for future events) once problems with fluid overload have been adequately treated. This approach, however, fails to recognize that the underlying progression of cardiac dysfunction caused by remodeling of the heart will continue and that this patient remains at high risk for future morbidity and mortality despite adequate treatment of the signs and symptoms of congestion.

Heart failure is a syndrome that can be caused by a variety of conditions that result in damage to the myocardium. These include myocardial infarction (MI), long-standing pressure or volume overload, myocyte damage caused by a viral infection, and damage caused by replacement of normal myocardium by infiltrative diseases, such as amyloidosis. Regardless of the cause, however, both the systemic response to altered cardiac function and the structural changes (and cellular processes) that develop within the heart itself in response to the initial injury are remarkably consistent. Thus, a characteristic of heart failure is that damage to the heart or prolonged increases in loading conditions result in a prototypic systemic and local cardiac neurohormonal response.

Abnormalities in Cardiac Function

The diagnosis of heart failure on the basis of systolic dysfunction implies an abnormality in the pumping capacity of the heart. If mechanical problems (ie, with cardiac filling or emptying [caused by valvular or pericardial disease] or movement of blood within the heart [on the basis of intracardiac shunting]) are excluded, the basis of this abnormality resides in an inability of the myo-cardium to generate adequate amounts of force with each contraction. Thus, heart failure is characterized by abnormal shortening of individual sarcomeres, which may be further worsened by abnormalities in the interstitium or extracellular matrix (ECM) of the heart. Conditions that can result in abnormal cardiac sarcomere shortening are summarized in Table 9-1, which is based on an excellent review of the subject by Braunwald and Bristow.[1]

An abnormality in energy metabolism refers to an inability of the heart to generate adequate energy within the myocytes, resulting in compromised shortening of the contractile units (sarcomeres). This may result from a variety of causes, including the effects of myocardial ischemia, presence of hypertrophy, reduction of high-energy creatine phosphate stores in the failing heart, mitochondrial abnormalities, and reduced activity of critical enzymes, such as creatine kinase. In all of these cases, the external work performed by the heart is compromised, while energy consumption remains in the normal or nearly normal range. Thus, the efficiency of cardiac function in the failing heart is abnormal.

In heart failure, the pattern of expression of several genes within the heart is altered.[2] Most commonly, the changes in gene expression seen in the failing heart seem to recapitulate the pattern seen during early development of the organism. This transition involves both quantitative changes in gene expression and changes in the expressed isoform of genes encoding important structural and functional proteins in the heart. The changes in gene expression in the failing heart have been termed a *reversion to the fetal gene pattern* because many of the changes are similar to those seen during early development.

Abnormalities in excitation-contraction coupling have also been identified in the failing heart. In the end-stage failing human heart, prolongation of the calcium transient and increased diastolic calcium concentrations have been

Table 9-1: Cellular Basis of Cardiac Failure[1]

- Abnormalities in energy metabolism
  - Relative subendocardial myocardial ischemia
  - Reduced high-energy (eg, creatine phosphate) stores
  - Mitochondrial abnormalities
  - Reduced creatine kinase activity

- Alteration in expression or activity of contractile proteins (ie, reversion to the 'fetal gene pattern')
  - Alterations in myosin heavy chain, troponin T, and myosin light chain-I

- Abnormalities in excitation-contraction coupling
  - Prolongation of intracellular Ca^+ transient
  - Increased diastolic Ca^+ concentrations

- Cytoskeletal abnormalities
  - Excessive microtubular polymerization
  - Increased cytoskeletal proteins (eg, tubulin, dystrophin)
  - Decreased cytoskeletal proteins (eg, α-actinin, titin)
  - Cytoskeletal gene mutations in dystrophin, desmin, sarcoglycans, and laminin A and C

- Alterations in β-adrenergic signaling

reported. These abnormalities are associated with the altered expression of genes for molecules such as sarcoplasmic reticular ATPase (SERCA) and its regulatory protein, phospholamban, both of which play an important role in the regulation of intracellular calcium concentrations.

Abnormally low expression of the transsarcolemmal Na^+/Ca^{2+} transporter, which helps remove calcium from the myocyte, has also been reported in heart failure and may result in similar effects on intracellular calcium fluxes.

A variety of cytoskeletal proteins, such as dystrophin, laminin, actinin, titin, and myomesin, play a role in this process, and several mutations in cytoskeletal genes have been shown to be involved in the pathogenesis of dilated cardiomyopathy in human patients.

In addition, there is evidence that alterations in β-adrenergic receptor signal transduction play an important role in the pathogenesis of heart failure. Multiple signaling abnormalities have been implicated in this process, including down-regulation of the β_1-adrenergic receptor on cardiac myocytes. The net effect is reduction in cardiac reserve and impairment of exercise capacity in heart failure patients.

Compensatory Mechanisms

The compensatory mechanisms that develop in the setting of heart failure are outlined in Table 9-2. Generally, they are activated as a means of compensating for a reduction in arterial perfusion pressure. They are usually best suited to providing short-term support for the cardiovascular system during periods of acute stress, since they serve the useful purpose of augmenting cardiac output and maintaining arterial pressure.

It is tempting to consider that these mechanisms may have developed during evolution as means of protection from decreased perfusion pressure caused by dehydration and blood loss. However, the sustained activation of these compensatory mechanisms in response to diminished cardiac output or arterial perfusion pressure caused by cardiac dysfunction is now recognized to have long-term consequences that are mostly deleterious. An example of this is the retention of salt and water that develops in response to a reduction in cardiac output and arterial perfu-

Table 9-2: Compensatory Mechanisms to Support the Failing Heart

Mechanism	Beneficial Effect
Immediate	
Salt/water retention	Increased intravascular volume resulting in increased CO and BP
Peripheral vasoconstriction	Increased venous return to the heart and augmented BP
Increased heart rate	Increased CO
Increased myo-cardial contractility	Increased CO
Long-term	
Myocardial hypertrophy	Increased force generation caused by an increased number of contractile units (ie, sarcomeres) Normalization of wall stress
Chamber dilation	Increased stroke volume

BP = blood pressure
CO = cardiac output

sion pressure. Initially, this results in an expansion of intracardiac volumes, which serves to increase cardiac output. However, this volume expansion also leads to worsening signs and symptoms of congestion and to an increased load on the heart. The resultant increase in wall stress, as we shall see later in this chapter, promotes adverse changes in cardiac structure that result in progressive deterioration in cardiac function.[3]

Deleterious Consequence
Increased wall stress
Pulmonary and systemic congestion
Increased wall stress
Pulmonary congestion
Increased myocardial oxygen consumption
Increased myocardial oxygen consumption
Abnormalities in structural and functional
proteins within the myocyte
Energy supply/demand mismatch
Increased fibrosis
Increased risk of arrhythmias[4]
Increased wall stress
2° valvular insufficiency

Cardiac Remodeling

In response to myocardial injury or to prolonged increases in pressure and/or volume load, the heart undergoes a prototypic series of changes in structure now commonly referred to as *cardiac remodeling*.[5] In this process (Table 9-3), eccentric hypertrophy of the myocardium develops, so there is an increase in both muscle mass and chamber volume of the left ventricle. Increased deposi-

Table 9-3: Characteristics of Cardiac Remodeling

1. Initiated by damage to the heart, such as myocardial injury or increased pressure or volume load

2. Often continues even after resolution of initiating event

3. Tends to progress over time

4. Results in increased cardiac chamber volumes and muscle mass (eccentric hypertrophy), as well as increased extracellular matrix deposition

tion of fibrous tissue in the ECM and alterations in the collagen characteristics also occur. The net effect of these changes is a progressive deterioration in both systolic and diastolic function of the heart.[6] Cardiac remodeling often continues well after the initiating event has resolved. Thus, even in the absence of continued or repetitive insults to the heart, remodeling may progress in an insidious manner, accounting for the all-too-common occurrence of heart failure as the first indication of a long-standing process that has resulted in extensive cardiac dysfunction.

The process of cardiac remodeling has been recognized in the post-MI population for some time, and most of our understanding of the clinical characteristics of cardiac remodeling comes from this population.[7,8] For many years, researchers have known that patients who experience large MIs or who have substantial amounts of myocardial damage because of repeated episodes of injury are at high risk for cardiac remodeling. Initially, remodeling involves primarily the infarct zone, in which necrotic myocardium is replaced by scar tissue. However, even during this early phase, there is evidence that structural changes also occur in the noninfarcted segments of the heart. Activation of matrix metalloproteinases (MMPs), a family of proteolytic enzymes, occurs and results in ventricular dilatation caused by breakdown of the ECM of the heart.[9] Later, further dilatation and hypertrophy of these noninfarcted segments occur so that what started as a discrete area of injury caused by an infarction progresses to a global process involving virtually all segments of the left ventricle.

The impact of remodeling on the clinical course is substantial.[10] Increases in ventricular volumes are associated with an increased risk of future cardiac events, including onset of heart failure, hospitalization, and death. Whereas hypertrophy was once considered a beneficial compensatory response, the adverse consequences of hypertrophy in the remodeling heart have now become apparent. A study of patients in the Studies of Left Ventricular Dysfunction (SOLVD) trials and registry followed the clinical course of patients with heart failure over a 12-month period.[11] Patients with an LV mass above the median value for the group had nearly a twofold increase in the likelihood of experiencing a cardiovascular event compared to patients whose mass was below the median value. Interestingly, the effect of increased mass on risk of future events was independent of the level of LVEF. Patients with a myocardial mass above the median value for the group continued to be at a greater risk for mortality or cardiovascular hospitalization regardless of whether their ejection fraction was above or below 0.35. These findings implicate increases in myocardial mass as a negative prognostic factor in heart failure with either preserved or depressed LVEF.

Although the connections between cardiac remodeling and abnormalities in contractile dysfunction are complex, the mechanisms involved are beginning to be elucidated.[12] Many of the pathways activated in the course of the development of cardiac hypertrophy also play a role in the development of myocardial dysfunction.[13] These include abnormalities in calcium handling, abnormal myocardial energetics, and induction of the fetal gene program. Increased amounts of ECM are also found in the remodeled hypertrophic heart and appear to play a particularly important role in patients with advanced systolic dysfunction. In a study of end-stage human ischemic cardiomyopathy, Beltrami et al found that approximately two thirds of the fibrous tissue found in the remodeling heart was located outside of the regions of previous MI.[14] Since fibrosis can impair both systolic and diastolic function of the heart, it seems likely that excess deposition of ECM in the remodeling heart is an important contributor to the progression of heart failure in this group.

Myocyte Apoptosis

As the heart remodels, there is evidence that a progressive loss of cardiac myocytes over time contributes to deterioration in cardiac function.[15,16] While myocyte death caused by myocardial ischemia and toxic effects of neurohormonal agents, such as norepinephrine and angiotensin II (Ang II), appears to be involved in this process, there is evidence that myocyte loss caused by other factors may also play a role. Specifically, a growing body of evidence from experimental animal models and from human patients suggests that cardiac cell death caused by apoptosis occurs after MI and as LV dysfunction progresses. Apoptosis is an active process about which a great deal has been learned over the past decade. Some of the important characteristics of this type of programmed cell death are summarized in Table 9-4.

The causes of myocyte apoptosis in the heart appear to be diverse. Factors that can trigger apoptosis have been identified in various experimental animal models and in cell culture experiments; some of the most important ones are listed in Table 9-5. Evidence of apoptosis has been obtained in human hearts from patients with ischemic as well as nonischemic cardiomyopathies. Researchers esti-

Table 9-4: Characteristics of Apoptosis

- Active, precisely regulated, energy-requiring process
- Orchestrated by a genetic program
- Plays a crucial role in regulating proliferating cell populations in adult tissues and in normal tissue development

Adapted from Sabbah, *Cardiovasc Res* 2000;45:704-712.[15]

Table 9-5: Causes of Cardiomyocyte Apoptosis

- Free oxygen radicals
- Angiotensin II
- Hypoxia
- Cytokines (ie, tumor necrosis factor-α)
- Calcium overload
- Norepinephrine

mate that apoptosis may result in the loss of 1% to 5% of cardiomyocytes each year in the failing human heart, a figure that, if correct, may well explain many aspects of the progressive nature of heart failure. Future heart failure therapies may be directed toward trying to block further worsening in cardiac function by inhibiting myocyte apoptosis. However, this issue is complicated by the fact that apoptosis is an important protective mechanism to help control unrestricted cell growth, and systemic blockade of this process would likely result in an increased risk of malignancies.

Table 9-6: Causes of Cardiac Remodeling

Hemodynamic Factors
- Pressure overload
- Volume overload

Neurohormonal Factors
- Angiotensin II
- Catecholamines
- Cytokines such as tumor necrosis factor-α
- Endothelin
- Aldosterone

Causes of Cardiac Remodeling

Much work has been carried out over the years in identifying the causes of cardiac remodeling. The major factors involved in the pathogenesis of remodeling are outlined in Table 9-6. The effects of either pressure load or volume load in causing structural changes in the heart have been recognized for some time. Both situations result in an increase in wall stress. However, although both initiate remodeling, the pattern that develops is somewhat different in each instance.

Pressure overload, such as occurs with hypertension or aortic stenosis, results in the development of concentric hypertrophy. In contrast, volume overload that occurs with conditions such as aortic or mitral regurgitation produces eccentric hypertrophy of the left ventricle. Although there is an increase in muscle mass in each of these types of hypertrophy, dilatation of the ventricle only accompanies volume overload. In pure pressure overload, the size of the ventricle does not increase at least until systolic dysfunction develops and the ventricle begins to fail. The remodeling that accompanies either pressure or volume overload is very much a compensatory response that enables the heart to accommodate changes in loading conditions and still maintain relatively normal function for an extended period. However, if the stimulus for continued growth and remodeling persists, cardiac function begins to deteriorate and heart failure ensues. The reasons for this are related to changes in cardiac cell phenotype that develop in the hypertrophic heart; myocardial oxygen supply-demand mismatches; and the adverse consequences of increased deposition of ECM within the heart. As stated previously, the presence of increased myocardial mass in heart failure patients with either preserved or impaired LV systolic function is an important negative prognostic risk factor.

Neurohormonal agents play a critical role in the remodeling process.[17] Although many neurohormonal systems are activated during the development of heart failure, the effects of Ang II, norepinephrine (NE), endothelin (ET), aldosterone, and proinflammatory cytokines (such as tumor necrosis factor-α [TNF-α]) appear to have the most important effects on the remodeling process (Table 9-7). The central position of neurohormonal activation in the pathogenesis of heart failure is outlined in Figure 9-2.

Generally, the effects of the various neurohormonal agents activated in the failing heart tend to work in a synergistic fashion to initiate the compensatory changes outlined earlier in this chapter. The early effects of neurohormonal activation, such as salt and water retention and peripheral vasoconstriction, tend to increase both the pressure and the volume loads on the heart. If sustained over time, this load increase will stimulate remodeling. However, many of the agents are also able to promote remodeling by their direct stimulation of either growth or activation of heart cells. In cardiomyocytes, neurohormonal agents promote cell hypertrophy and expression of the fetal gene pattern, with a resultant alteration in several important myocyte proteins. In fibroblasts, neurohormonal activation increases cell replication, migration, and pro-

Table 9-7: Effects of Neurohormonal Agents on Cardiac Remodeling

Agent	Effect on Cardiac Load
Ang II	Increases salt/water retention
	Increases peripheral resistance
NE	Increases salt/water retention
	Increases peripheral resistance
ET	Increases salt/water retention
TNF-α	

Ang II = angiotensin II
ECM = extracellular matrix
ET = endothelin
MMPs = matrix metalloproteinases

duction of ECM proteins, such as fibronectin and collagen.[18] Thus, neurohormonal agents have direct (growth-related) as well as indirect (increased load) effects that promote the remodeling process.

Effect on Cardiac Cells/ECM	Effect on Other Neurohormonal Systems
Stimulates myocyte hypertrophy Stimulates fibroblasts to produce ECM Increases production of TIMPs that block ECM breakdown	Stimulates prejunctional receptors on adrenergic nerves to release NE Stimulates cardiac cells to release ET
Stimulates myocyte hypertrophy Stimulates fibroblasts to produce ECM	Stimulates release of renin activity from the kidney
Stimulates myocyte hypertrophy Stimulates fibroblasts to produce ECM	
Stimulates myocyte hypertrophy Activates MMPs that break down ECM Depresses myocardial contractility	Upregulates expression of Ang II receptors

NE = norepinephrine
TIMPs = tissue inhibitors of metalloproteinases
TNF = tumor necrosis factor

Evidence suggests that a great deal of crosstalk occurs between the neurohormonal systems, so activation of one system often results in enhanced activation of other systems. For example, one effect of NE is stimu-

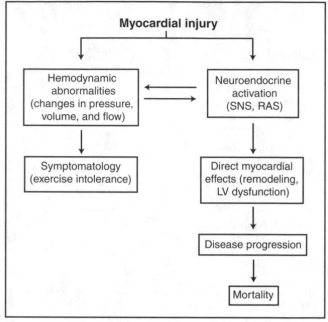

Figure 9-2: Heart failure pathophysiology. LV = left ventricular, RAS = renin-angiotensin system, SNS = sympathetic nervous system. From Packer, *J Am Coll Cardiol* 1992;20:248-254.[17]

lating the release of renin activity from the juxtaglomerular apparatus of the kidney. Similarly, proinflammatory cytokines that are released in the post-MI heart act to increase angiotensin receptor density on cardiac fibroblasts, an effect that enhances the growth-promoting effects of Ang II on these cells.[19] However, not all of the neurohormonal agents that are increased in the failing heart promote cardiac remodeling. Elevated wall stress within the heart increases production and release of factors such as atrial natriuretic peptide (ANP) and brain natriuretic peptide (BNP), which have both vasodilatory and diuretic properties. The natriuretic peptides appear to inhibit release of growth-promoting neurohormones, such as ET, and they act directly to inhibit growth and activation of cardiac cells. Thus, they tend to regulate the adverse consequences of other agents that are activated locally and systemically, such as the renin-angiotensin and sympathetic nervous systems. Unfortunately, there is an imbalance between the factors that promote remodeling and those that inhibit it, so although the natriuretic peptides may modulate the process somewhat, the net effect of neurohormonal activation is to stimulate cardiac growth.

Systemic neurohormonal activation is a consequence of hemodynamic perturbations that cause a reduction in perfusion pressure, while local activation of systems within the heart can be initiated either by altered hemodynamics (usually associated with increased ventricular filling pressures) or in response to myocardial damage.[20] Systemic neurohormonal activation begins early after damage to the heart occurs. After an MI, there is evidence of widespread neurohormonal activation that probably develops as a way to maintain perfusion pressure for vital organs.[21] With resolution of the acute event, some of these systemic factors become quiescent. However, activation of systems (eg, the intracardiac renin-angiotensin system) also occurs within the heart.

Persistent activation of neurohormonal systems, both systemically and locally within the heart, results in increased load and sustained stimulation of cardiac cells, both of which drive the remodeling process. Results from a survey of neurohormones sampled from the blood of patients with LV dysfunction in the SOLVD program are helpful in explaining the pattern and importance of neurohormonal activation in the development of heart failure. Patients enrolled in SOLVD had evidence of LV dysfunction, manifested by an EF <0.35. Subjects without evidence of symptomatic heart failure were enrolled

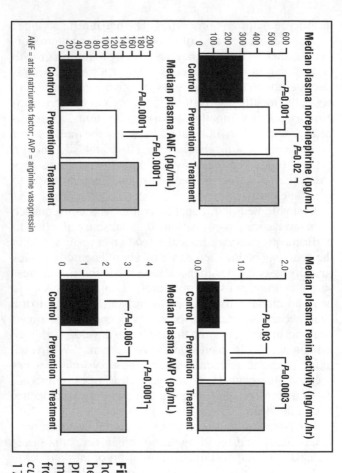

Figure 9-3: Neurohormonal activation in heart failure (SOLVD prevention and treatment trials). Adapted from Francis et al, *Circulation* 1990;82: 1724-1729.[22]

ANF = atrial natriuretic factor; AVP = arginine vasopressin

in the prevention arm of the study, while patients with the usual signs and symptoms of heart failure were enrolled in the treatment arm. As depicted in Figure 9-3, evidence showed an increase in the levels of the neurohormones sampled in the asymptomatic prevention arm patients.[22] In the symptomatic treatment arm patients, further activation of these systems became evident. The results of this study provide evidence that neurohormonal activation precedes the development of overt heart failure. Since these factors tend to promote growth, these findings suggest that early neurohormonal activation plays a causative role in the remodeling process. The results also show that as heart failure progresses, further neurohormonal activation occurs, indicating an intensification of the process.

Perhaps the most persuasive evidence that neurohormonal activation causes remodeling comes from a substantial body of evidence from large-scale clinical trials in which neurohormonal blocking agents, such as angiotensin-converting enzyme (ACE) inhibitors and β-blockers, were given to patients with heart failure. These studies are reviewed extensively in the respective chapters dealing with these agents. However, the results demonstrate that neurohormonal blocking agents are associated with inhibition of the remodeling process.[5,10,23] This effect appears to be related to the favorable impact that these agents have on the clinical course of heart failure patients and provides the basis for the use of drugs, such as ACE inhibitors and β-blockers, for the treatment of heart failure.

References

1.   Braunwald E, Bristow MR: Congestive heart failure: fifty years of progress. *Circulation* 2000;102(suppl 4):IV14-IV23.

2.   Schwartz K, Carrier L, Mercadier JJ, et al: Molecular phenotype of the hypertrophied and failing myocardium. *Circulation* 1993;87(suppl 7):VII5-VII10.

3. Vasan RS, Larson MG, Benjamin EJ, et al: Left ventricular dilatation and the risk of congestive heart failure in people without myocardial infarction. *N Engl J Med* 1997;336:1350-1355.

4. Levy D, Anderson KM, Savage DD, et al: Risk of ventricular arrhythmias in left ventricular hypertrophy: the Framingham heart study. *Am J Cardiol* 1987;60:560-565.

5. Cohn JN, Ferrari R, Sharpe N: Cardiac remodeling—concepts and clinical implications: a consensus paper from an international forum on cardiac remodeling. On behalf of the International Forum on Cardiac Remodeling. *J Am Coll Cardiol* 2000;35:569-582.

6. Mercadier JJ: Progression from cardiac hypertrophy to heart failure. In: Hosenpud JD, Greenberg BH, eds. *Congestive Heart Failure. Pathophysiology, Diagnosis and Comprehensive Approach to Management*, 2nd ed. Philadelphia, Lippincott Williams and Wilkins, 2000, pp 41-65.

7. McKay RG, Pfeffer MA, Pasternak RC, et al: Left ventricular remodeling after myocardial infarction: a corollary to infarct expansion. *Circulation* 1986;74:693-702.

8. Sutton MG, Sharpe N: Left ventricular remodeling after myocardial infarction: pathophysiology and therapy. *Circulation* 2000; 101:2981-2988.

9. Weber KT: Extracellular matrix remodeling in heart failure: a role for de novo angiotensin II generation. *Circulation* 1997;96: 4065-4082.

10. St. John Sutton M, Pfeffer MA, Plappert T, et al: Quantitative two-dimensional echocardiographic measurements are major predicators of adverse cardiovascular events after acute myocardial infarction. The protective effects of captopril. *Circulation* 1994;89:68-75.

11. Quinones MA, Greenberg BH, Kopelen HA, et al: Echocardiographic predictors of clinical outcome in patients with left ventricular dysfunction enrolled in the SOLVD registry and trials: significance of left ventricular hypertrophy. Studies of Left Ventricular Dysfunction. *J Am Coll Cardiol* 2000;35:1237-1244.

12. Katz AM: The cardiomyopathy of overload: an unnatural growth response in the hypertrophied heart. *Ann Intern Med* 1994;121:363-371.

13. Hunter JJ, Chien KR: Signaling pathways for cardiac hypertrophy and failure. *N Engl J Med* 1999;341:1276-1283.

14. Beltrami CA, Finato N, Rocco M, et al: Structural basis of end-stage failure in ischemic cardiomyopathy in humans. *Circulation* 1994;89:151-163.

15. Sabbah HN: Apoptotic cell death in heart failure. *Cardiovasc Res* 2000;45:704-712.

16. Sabbah HN, Sharov VG, Goldstein S: Cell death, tissue hypoxia and the progression of heart failure. *Heart Fail Rev* 2000;5:131-138.

17. Packer M: The neurohormonal hypothesis: a theory to explain the mechanism of disease progression in heart failure. *J Am Coll Cardiol* 1992;20:248-254.

18. Sadoshima J, Izumo S: Molecular characterization of angiotensin II-induced hypertrophy of cardiac myocytes and hyperplasia of cardiac fibroblasts. Critical role of the AT_1 receptor subtype. *Circ Res* 1993;73:413-423.

19. Peng J, Gurantz D, Tran V, et al: Tumor necrosis factor-alpha-induced AT1 receptor upregulation enhances angiotension II-mediated cardiac fibroblast responses that favor fibrosis. *Circ Res* 2002;91:1119-1126.

20. Schrier RW, Abraham WT: Hormones and hemodynamics in heart failure. *N Engl J Med* 1999;341:577-585.

21. Rouleau JL, De Champlain J, Klein M, et al: Activation of neurohumoral systems in postinfarction left ventricular dysfunction. *J Am Coll Cardiol* 1993;22:390-398.

22. Francis GS, Benedict C, Johnstone DE, et al: Comparison of neuroendocrine activation in patients with left ventricular dysfunction with and without congestive heart failure. A substudy of the Studies of Left Ventricular Dysfunction (SOLVD). *Circulation* 1990;82:1724-1729.

23. Greenberg B, Quinones MA, Koilpillai C, et al: Effects of long-term enalapril therapy on cardiac structure and function in patients with left ventricular dysfunction. Results of the SOLVD echocardiography substudy. *Circulation* 1995;91:2573-2581.

Chapter **10**

Diagnosis and Evaluation of Heart Failure

Heart failure, a complex clinical syndrome diagnosed by the presence of a symptom complex derived from impaired cardiac function, may be either acute or chronic. The 'classic' presentation of acute, severe heart failure evokes an image of a patient with pink, frothy pulmonary edema fluid, diffuse pulmonary rales, and overt cardiogenic shock. However, identical hemodynamic measurements without extreme symptoms or physical examination signs are commonly found in the patient with chronic heart failure, reflecting a slow and insidious onset. Consequently, while the acute presentation is easily recognized, classic symptoms of chronic heart failure (dyspnea, fatigue) are frequently misinterpreted in clinical practice. This chapter focuses on the diagnosis and evaluation of the patient with chronic heart failure.

Heart failure is a preventable disease. Early identification and treatment of left ventricular dysfunction (LVD) saves lives. Therefore, patients at risk for the development of heart failure should be assessed periodically for attributable symptoms. Common independent risk factors for chronic heart failure include aging, atherosclerotic coronary disease, diabetes, hypertension, LV hypertrophy, and obesity. Clinicians should note that impaired LV function may, in fact, be asymptomatic, although slowly progressive symptoms may be rationalized as a 'normal' consequence of aging or attributed to poor physical conditioning.

The American College of Cardiology and American Heart Association Task Force of Practice Guidelines have created a novel four-stage grading system for chronic heart failure (Table 10-1).[1] These guidelines have been officially endorsed by the Heart Failure Society of America and the International Society of Heart and Lung Transplantation. The staging system focuses on heart failure as a progressive disorder rather than as a symptomatic disease. The evolution and progression of heart failure are characterized by four stages of disease progression, starting with asymptomatic patients at risk. In these patients, left ventricular dysfunction arises from myocardial injury or stress. Once sufficient injury has occurred, the process of heart failure generally continues, even in the absence of further insult to the heart. The mechanism of this progression, known as *cardiac remodeling*, manifests as a change in the geometry of the left ventricle, including chamber dilation, increasing sphericity, and hypertrophy.[2] These morphologic changes increase hemodynamic stress on the walls of the failing heart, further depress mechanical performance, and promote continued remodeling. Not all patients progress sequentially through these stages, although most do. This staging system allows the use of specific treatments targeted at each stage for the purpose of reducing morbidity and mortality.

Symptoms

Heart failure is the symptomatic manifestation of the heart's inability to generate sufficient cardiac output to meet the metabolic needs of body tissues without or despite intracardiac hemodynamic perturbation. Symptoms commonly observed in chronic heart failure patients are typically categorized as *congestive* or *low cardiac output* (Table 10-2), but they may coexist regardless of category.[1,3] The adjective *congestive* is most appropriate when symptoms or signs of systemic or pulmonary fluid volume overload exist.

Table 10-1: American College of Cardiology/American Heart Association Stages of Heart Failure

Stage	Description
A	Patients at high risk of developing heart failure because of the presence of conditions that are strongly associated with the development of heart failure. Such patients have no identified structural or functional abnormalities of the pericardium, myocardium, or cardiac valves and have never shown signs or symptoms of heart failure.
B	Patients with structural heart disease that is strongly associated with the development of heart failure but who have never shown signs or symptoms of heart failure.
C	Patients who have current or prior symptoms of heart failure associated with underlying structural heart disease.
D	Patients with advanced structural heart disease and marked symptoms of heart failure at rest despite maximal medical therapy and who require specialized interventions.

Although it is a common misperception, the diagnosis of chronic heart failure does not indicate the underlying etiology or nature of cardiac dysfunction (systolic vs diastolic).[4,5] Symptoms consistent with chronic heart

Examples

Systemic hypertension; coronary artery disease; diabetes mellitus; history of cardiotoxic drug therapy or alcohol abuse; personal history of rheumatic fever; family history of cardiomyopathy

Left ventricular hypertrophy or fibrosis; left ventricular dilatation or hypocontractility; asymptomatic valvular heart disease; previous myocardial infarction

Dyspnea or fatigue caused by left ventricular systolic dysfunction; ventricular systolic dysfunction; asymptomatic patients who are undergoing treatment for prior symptoms of heart failure

Patients who are frequently hospitalized for heart failure and cannot be safely discharged from the hospital; patients awaiting heart transplantation; patients at home receiving continuous intravenous support for symptom relief; patients being supported with a mechanical circulatory assist device; patients in a hospice setting for the management of heart failure symptoms

failure are often observed in noncardiac conditions, such as primary pulmonary hypertension and cor pulmonale. The differential diagnosis of heart failure is shown in Table 10-3.

Table 10-2: Common Symptoms of Chronic Heart Failure

Congestive
- Dyspnea (rest or exertional)
- Paroxysmal nocturnal dyspnea
- Abdominal or epigastric discomfort
- Nausea
- Early satiety or anorexia
- Pedal/leg edema
- Sleep disturbance (anxiety or air hunger)
- Orthopnea
- Cough (recumbent or exertional)
- Abdominal bloating (ascites)
- Weight gain (rapid)
- Chest tightness or discomfort

Low Cardiac Output
- Easy fatigability
- Nausea
- Early satiety or anorexia
- Poor energy level or endurance
- Weight loss, unexplained
- Impaired concentration or memory
- Sleep disturbance (Cheyne-Stokes respiration)
- Malaise
- Decreased exercise tolerance
- Muscle wasting or weakness
- Daytime oliguria with recumbent nocturia

Table 10-3: Differential Diagnosis of Chronic Heart Failure

Dyspnea +/- Edema

- Pulmonary parenchymal disease, chronic obstructive or interstitial
- Pulmonary thromboembolic disease
- Cor pulmonale
- Pulmonary venous occlusive disease
- Primary pulmonary hypertension
- Other secondary pulmonary hypertension
- Exertional asthma
- Severe anemia
- Mitral stenosis
- Neuromuscular disease
- Constrictive pericarditis
- Metabolic causes (acidosis)
- Restrictive infiltrative or hypertrophic myocardial disease
- Atrial myxoma

Edema +/- Dyspnea

- Nephrotic syndrome
- Cirrhosis
- Venous insufficiency
- Combined vascular insufficiency (arterial and venous)
- Lymphedema
- Adverse medication effect (vasodilators)

**Table 10-4: New York Heart Association
Functional Classification
of Chronic Heart Failure**

Class	Symptoms
I	No perceived limitation of physical activity
II A/B	Symptoms with moderate physical exertion
III A/B	Symptoms with low levels of physical exertion (ie, those for activities of daily living)
IV	Resting symptoms

A = early stage; B = late stage

Despite well-known subjective limitations, symptoms are traditionally classified according to the New York Heart Association (NYHA) Classification (Table 10-4). NYHA Class I patients have no perceived limitation of physical activity. In NYHA Class II patients, physical exertion produces heart failure symptoms (eg, fatigue, dyspnea). NYHA Class III patients are comfortable at rest but develop heart failure symptoms with low levels of activity, such as those required for the activities of daily living. NYHA Class IV patients experience resting symptoms. Classes II and III are often difficult to distinguish and have been further subcategorized into NYHA II A/B and III A/B, reflecting early vs late symptom manifestations in each stage.[1,3]

In assessing NYHA symptom class, clinicians should try to maintain a frame of reference to the typical activities of an age- and gender-matched normal individual. In each patient, symptom classification is subject to fluctuation. The NYHA classification describing the patient's baseline *com-*

pensated state is most useful for the purpose of titration of medical therapy and for determining prognosis. Despite its limitations, NYHA symptom classification is still useful as a surrogate predictor of clinical outcome. Generally, patients with NYHA Class IV symptoms have significantly worsened survival (40% to 60% annual mortality risk) compared with NYHA Class I/IIA patients (5% to 10% annual mortality risk).[1,3,6,7] Interestingly, there is no correlation between symptom class and LV ejection fraction (LVEF).

Medical History and Physical Examination

In a patient with symptoms of chronic heart failure, the medical history and physical examination should focus on determining the etiology of cardiac dysfunction and other factors contributing to symptom precipitation. In many cases, treatment of the initiating disease process may improve cardiac function.

Coronary Artery Disease

In the United States, 60% to 75% of patients in clinical trials of heart failure and systolic LVD have underlying ischemic cardiomyopathy.[2,7,8] Patients with both heart failure and risk factors for coronary artery disease (CAD) should be evaluated for the presence of CAD, as revascularization may be appropriate.

Hypertension

Hypertension is a risk factor for the development of CAD, but it is also an independent risk factor for the development of heart failure.[9-11] In patient populations with heart failure and preserved systolic LV function, a history of hypertension is extremely common. A history of hypertension is also predominant in the subpopulations of women, African-Americans, and the elderly with heart failure.[12-17] Patients on chronic antihypertensive therapy with long-standing inadequate resting or exertional blood pressure control, those with recorded systolic blood pressures >200 mm Hg, and those who have been treated for hypertensive urgencies or crises are likely to have hypertensive cardiomyopathy (increased LV mass and wall thickness, reflecting myocardial hypertrophy). In late stages, hypertensive heart failure can result in progressive LV chamber dilation, wall thinning, and impairment of systolic function.

Endocrinopathy

Diabetes. Cardiomyopathy in association with long-standing diabetes has been described (excluding CAD), although typically in association with additional end-organ damage.[18-20] Diabetic amyloid deposition in the myocardium may initially contribute to diastolic myocardial relaxation abnormalities, followed by systolic ventricular impairment. Additionally, uncontrolled diabetes promotes decompensation of chronic heart failure related to hyperosmolar stress and increased infection risk. Oxidative stress induced by diabetes appears to promote cardiac progenitor cell aging, senescence, and apoptosis.[20]

Thyroid disease. Asymptomatic or symptomatic thyroid conditions related to either hypo- or hyperthyroidism can induce or exacerbate underlying myocardial dysfunction, mediated by isoform alterations in myocardial myosin.[19,21]

Growth hormone excess, pheochromocytoma, hyperaldosteronism, Cushing's syndrome. These conditions are fairly rare, but treatable.

Recent Pregnancy

Heart failure occurring within months after the delivery of a child in a woman with no prior history of heart disease, preeclampsia, or other identified etiology of cardiomyopathy is likely to be caused by peripartum cardiomyopathy. The incidence is fairly uncommon, occurring in about one of 3,189 live births.[22] In this setting, the natural history is similar to that of idiopathic cardiomyopathy.[19]

Family History

Researchers estimate that nearly 10% to 15% of heart failure patients may have a family history of cardiomyopathy. A family history of sudden unexplained (cardiac) death should, therefore, be sought in all patients. The most detailed genetic linkages reflect variants of hypertrophic cardiomyopathy. Additional inheritable cardiomyopathies, such as hemochromocytosis or muscular dystrophies, should be considered in the appropriate setting.[19]

Substance Abuse

A careful history of the quantity of alcohol consumed and the frequency of consumption should be obtained from each patient. Generally, chronic consumption of ethanol for a prolonged duration (typically several years) and the exclusion of other causes are required to attribute a heart failure diagnosis to alcoholic cardiomyopathy.[3,19,23] The degree of myocardial apoptosis is similar between alcoholics and persons with long-standing hypertension.[23] Cardiomyopathy has also been observed in association with chronic amphetamine and/or cocaine use. These agents may cause direct myocardial toxicity or affect ventricular function through either small- or large-vessel CAD or vascular dysfunction. Current and former intravenous drug users may present with progressive valvular heart disease from prior infectious endocarditis. Patients with a lifestyle risk of intravenous substance abuse are also at risk for hepatitis C viral infection, which has been associated with a dilated cardiomyopathy.[19]

Drugs and Toxins

Chemotherapeutic agents. Doxorubicin (Adriamycin®) and other anthracyclines, cyclophosphamide (Cytoxan®, Neosar®), and several other chemotherapeutic agents may cause acute (peak bolus dose) toxic myocardial damage. Cumulative dose toxicity represents a more chronic form of injury and is infrequent with anthracyclines at doses less than 400 to 450 mg/m^2. However, subclinical myocardial injury that occurs during drug administration may result in progressive ventricular remodeling and late-onset heart failure months to years later.[1,3,19] Certain risk factors (advanced age, concomitant mediastinal irradiation, preexisting myocardial disease) increase the likelihood of myocardial toxicity. Chemotherapy-related cardiomyopathy, however, represents a diagnosis of exclusion when heart failure is of late onset. In addition to direct myocardial cellular injury, an eosinophilic myocarditis has been reported in association with interleukin-2 (IL-2) administration.[24]

Inflammatory myocardial disease. Several common pharmacologic agents have potential cardiotoxic effects (eg, high-dose catecholamine administration). Other drugs have been associated with either direct toxic or hypersensitivity (allergic) eosinophilic myocarditis. Sulfa- or sulfur-containing drugs predominate, although others include such commonly used agents as quinidine (Quinidex®, Quinaglute®), hydralazine (Apresoline®), amitriptyline (eg, Elavil®), spironolactone (Aldactone®), acetazolamide (eg, Diamox®), isoniazid (eg, Laniazid®), penicillin, amphotericin B (Fungizone®), phenothiazines, carbamazepine (eg, Tegretol®), and phenytoin (eg, Dilantin®).[1,3]

Negatively inotropic medications. Agents such as calcium-channel blockers, (full-dose) β-blockers, and most antiarrhythmic drugs that depress cardiac function may precipitate heart failure symptoms. However, this probably represents an exacerbation of preexisting or subclinical cardiac dysfunction of another etiology.

Medications causing fluid retention. Institution of agents that promote avid sodium and water retention may also precipitate congestive heart failure symptoms in patients with preexisting or subclinical cardiac dysfunction. These drugs include, but are not limited to, nonsteroidal anti-inflammatory drugs (NSAIDs), corticosteroids, COX-2 inhibitors, peripherally acting α-blockers for the treatment of benign prostatic hypertrophy, hormone replacement or modulation therapy, and several of the newer glitazone class of insulin-sensitizing drugs.[1,3,25] Over-the-counter or naturoceutical products may also contribute to water retention.

Other toxins. Lead, arsenic, and cobalt are toxic metals that can cause progressive and dose-related myocardial dysfunction when consumed. Endogenous toxins that depress myocardial function are classically seen in uremia and sepsis (tumor necrosis factor-α).

Connective Tissue and Other Systemic Disorders

Patients with systemic lupus erythematosus, scleroderma, polymyositis, and other connective tissue disorders may develop an associated cardiomyopathy with heart failure.[1,3,19] In these conditions, as well as in granulomatous disorders (ie, sarcoidosis) and infiltrative disease (amyloidosis), the typical patient presents with heart failure and initially preserved systolic ventricular function.[11]

Myocarditis

Some forms of myocarditis are catastrophic in their initial presentation, such as fulminant viral myocarditis and giant cell myocarditis. More commonly, postviral myocarditis is characterized by a subacute onset, reflecting a gradual deterioration after resolution of the acute viral syndrome.[1,2,19] At least 20 viruses have been causally associated with clinical evidence of myocarditis, generally those causing upper respiratory or gastrointestinal syndromes. Heart failure caused by HIV-related cardiomyopathy is an uncommon presentation of HIV infection but is easily screened for in appropriate patients. Other infectious etiologies of myocarditis (eg, parasitic, chagasic, viral, rickettsial, bacterial, and fungal) are extremely uncommon.

Metabolic Deficiencies

Beriberi (thiamine deficiency) may appear in individuals on fad diets or on long-term, high-dose diuretics and in hospitalized patients receiving only salt or glucose replacement without proper nutritional support.[1,19] Inherited or acquired metabolic deficiencies (carnitine, coenzyme Q-10) are rare.

Hemoglobinopathies

Patients with certain hemoglobinopathies, such as thalassemia and sickle cell disease, who have undergone repeated transfusions can develop heart failure related to myocardial iron overload accompanying a high-output state derived from chronic anemia.[19]

High-Output States

Hyperthyroidism, severe chronic anemia, large intrinsic or iatrogenic arteriovenous shunts, Paget's disease, and sepsis may result in high-output failure.[19,21]

Valvular Heart Disease

Although this category represented the most common etiology of heart failure in the early Framingham studies, valvular disease is now more often a consequence of ventricular dilation than a cause. However, a history of rheumatic or other valvular disease can be important in defining the etiology of the patient's cardiac dysfunction, as the physical findings may be muted by low cardiac output or high filling pressures.

Idiopathic Etiology

When ventricular dysfunction presents without identifiable etiology or specific causative factor, the term *idiopathic cardiomyopathy* is generally used. This etiology represents approximately 10% to 20% of patient populations with heart failure.[1,3,6]

Physical Examination: Hemodynamic and Volume Assessment

Physical signs of chronic heart failure are often subtle and, like radiographic findings, have poor positive and negative predictive value in estimating intracardiac hemodynamics. For example, patients may have a marked elevation of pulmonary capillary wedge pressure (left atrial pressure) without manifesting pulmonary rales, if the hemodynamic perturbation was slowly achieved. However, while physical signs in chronic heart failure have diagnostic limitations, certain abnormalities have profound prognostic implications. For example, the presence of elevated jugular venous pressure, rales, and an S3 in a patient with chronic heart failure imply a much more adverse prognosis.

Common physical findings in chronic heart failure with correlative hemodynamic derangements are listed in Table 10-5.[4,5] Resting tachycardia is a frequent manifestation

Table 10-5: Physical Examination Findings and Typically Associated Hemodynamic Perturbations in Chronic Heart Failure

Reduced Cardiac Output

- Resting tachycardia
- Pulsus alternans
- Cachexia
- Cheyne-Stokes respiration (with or without apnea)
- Low carotid pulse volume
- Cool or vasoconstricted extremities
- Altered mentation (somnolence, confusion)

Volume and/or Diastolic Pressure Overload

- Jugular venous distention
- Abdominojugular reflux
- Ascites
- S3
- Hepatomegaly
- Pleural effusion
- Dependent edema
- Loud pulmonic closure sound
- Pulmonary rales

Nonspecific Hemodynamic Correlation

- Cardiomegaly
- S4
- Accessory respiratory muscle use
- Wheezing
- Subxiphoid impulse
- Abnormal apical impulse
- Tachypnea
- Parasternal lift

of the hyperadrenergic state, designed as an intrinsic compensatory mechanism to preserve resting cardiac output. A resting heart rate >120 to 130 beats/min may suggest tachycardia-induced cardiomyopathy. However, in most patients with heart failure, resting tachycardia represents a compensatory response to maintain cardiac output and tissue perfusion in the setting of clinical decompensation.

Venous Inspection

Marked jugular venous distention (>15 cm of water) or a lesser degree of elevation with Kussmaul's physiology (absence of an inspiratory pressure drop) indicates restrictive right heart filling.[5] This may reveal the etiology of cardiac dysfunction (restrictive/constrictive disease) or merely reflect severe biventricular failure with volume overload.[26] Massive jugular v-waves suggest severe tricuspid regurgitation and, therefore, either primary or secondary pulmonary hypertension. Abdominojugular reflux is frequently demonstrated in volume overload states. Hepatic enlargement or tenderness secondary to right heart congestion should be sought; hepatic pulsatility suggests significant tricuspid regurgitation.

Arterial Inspection

Carotid upstrokes should be assessed for delay, indicating hemodynamically significant aortic stenosis. Bifid and dynamic carotid pulsation may indicate hypertrophic cardiomyopathy. Carotid bruits or signs of peripheral arterial disease increase the likelihood of associated atherosclerotic CAD. Low-volume impulses are often palpated in a low cardiac output state. *Pulsus alternans* implies low cardiac output and severe systolic ventricular dysfunction.[5]

Peripheral Perfusion

Assessment or palpation of warm extremities with good capillary refill generally reflects an adequate resting cardiac output. Cool, vasoconstricted extremities with or without mild cyanosis imply significantly reduced cardiac output, with increased systemic vascular resistance as a compensatory mechanism to preserve vital organ perfusion.

Marked lower-extremity edema without an elevation in jugular venous pressure should prompt an evaluation for chronic venous insufficiency or thrombosis, hypoalbuminemia, or hepatic disease. In the setting of jugular distention, ascites disproportionate to lower-extremity edema may suggest restrictive/constrictive cardiomyopathy or severe tricuspid regurgitation.

Chest Palpation/Percussion

Chest palpation/percussion reveals the presence of cardiac enlargement by localizing the apical impulse. A forceful point of maximal impulse (PMI) with an S4 gallop suggests LV hypertrophy, while a parasternal heave typically suggests right ventricular hypertrophy and enlargement. A loud or palpable pulmonic closure sound may be heard in patients with pulmonary hypertension. An inferolaterally displaced PMI represents significant ventricular dilation and in the presence of a dyskinetic apical impulse is a sensitive, but not specific, finding of underlying ischemic cardiomyopathy. A displaced PMI accompanied by an S3 gallop is the most specific finding for systolic LVD.

Auscultation

Cardiac murmurs, including aortic stenosis, aortic regurgitation, mitral stenosis, and mitral regurgitation, may indicate a surgically remediable etiology of heart failure. However, an elevation in ventricular end-diastolic pressure or a reduced cardiac output may soften regurgitant and stenotic murmurs.[5] Auscultation of the lung fields seeks evidence of pleural effusion, rales, or wheezes (cardiac asthma). A more sensitive but subtle finding in chronic heart failure is limited inspiratory diaphragmatic descent, reflecting decreased lung compliance caused by an increase in interstitial lung water. Gallops can be variable and may derive from either the right or left ventricle. However, a left-sided S3 is classically associated with systolic ventricular dysfunction and impairment of early ventricular filling, which is more likely in LV volume overload. An S4 is more likely related to an increase in end-diastolic pressure/loading conditions with ventricular relaxation abnormality.

Diagnostic Evaluation

The clinical diagnosis of heart failure and its suspected pathophysiology must be confirmed by objective evaluation. All patients with symptoms or signs consistent with heart failure should undergo a formal assessment of cardiac function.[1,3] Specifically, the LVEF and wall motion should be evaluated by echocardiography with Doppler imaging or radionuclide ventriculography.[27-30] These testing modalities can also evaluate ventricular diastolic filling pattern and rate and, therefore, can indicate predominant systolic or diastolic dysfunction, or both. A diagnostic treatment algorithm emphasizing the importance of evaluation and treatment for underlying CAD is shown in Figure 10-1.

After confirming the diagnosis and character of ventricular dysfunction, the next step is to determine the etiology of chronic heart failure. When CAD is suspected, noninvasive stress testing for perfusion abnormalities or direct coronary angiography should be performed. In the absence of active or reversible ischemia, an assessment of myocardial viability should be considered, as reversible or treatable factors for ongoing myocardial injury must not be overlooked.[1,3]

The electrocardiogram (ECG) is not a useful screening tool for assessing either the presence or etiology of heart failure, but it should be obtained. Left atrial enlargement, atrial fibrillation, LV hypertrophy, old myocardial infarction, left bundle branch block, left axis deviation, and repolarization abnormalities are extremely common findings on ECG. A low QRS voltage or a pseudoinfarction pattern may direct attention to otherwise occult primary or secondary myocardial disease, such as amyloidosis.

Baseline two-view chest radiography should also be performed, as it provides information on general cardiac chamber size, great vessel enlargement or tortuosity, abnormal thoracic calcification, and concomitant lung parenchymal or vascular disease, including pulmonary

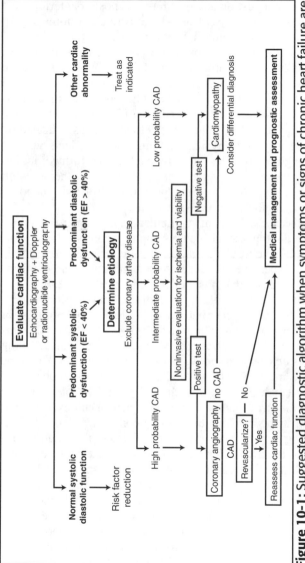

Figure 10-1: Suggested diagnostic algorithm when symptoms or signs of chronic heart failure are present. CAD = coronary artery disease; EF = ejection fraction.

venous congestion and pruning. The posteroanterior chest radiograph alone will not demonstrate cardiomegaly in the setting of isolated LV enlargement.

Additional testing commonly performed on patients with the clinical syndrome of heart failure includes a baseline screening laboratory assessment consisting of a standard chemistry profile with renal and hepatic function, a sensitive thyroid-stimulating hormone (TSH) assay, a complete blood count (CBC), and other blood tests, as indicated by the history and physical examination.[1,3] Patients without fasting lipid profiles should have them performed. In diabetic patients, measurement of glycosylated hemoglobin provides a sense of recent glycemic control, a risk factor in worsening heart failure symptoms.

Because significant ventricular dysfunction may produce few symptoms, and because symptoms consistent with heart failure have a substantial diagnostic differential, a simple yet inexpensive and accurate screening test that confirms or excludes a diagnosis of heart failure is appealing. Derived from ventricular myocardium, brain natriuretic peptide (BNP, or n-terminal pro-BNP) assays hold promise for this purpose.[31-34] An abnormal >100 pg/mL BNP level seems to be predictive of any perturbation in ventricular filling pressure or increased wall stress. However, BNP baseline levels increase with age and are >100 pg/mL in one out of four female patients older than 75 years. The role of BNP in the clinical evaluation and management of chronic heart failure patients remains to be more completely defined. BNP testing may be best used in cases where the diagnosis remains uncertain after the history, physical examination, and available conventional noninvasive diagnostic tests have been performed. For example, the assay may be particularly helpful in the rapid evaluation of acute dyspnea in the emergency department or urgent-care outpatient setting.[32] The role of BNP is being evaluated in screening high-risk populations, in monitoring response to medical therapy, or as an adjunct in estimating prognosis in chronic heart failure.[33,34]

Additional Useful Tests

Standard exercise stress testing (bicycle or treadmill) provides an objective assessment of a patient's functional exercise limitation and hemodynamic response to exercise. It also helps screen for evidence of exercise-induced arrhythmia or ischemia (angina); however, the ECG is typically nondiagnostic for ischemia in patients with heart failure caused by resting abnormalities or medication effects.

However, when combined with either echocardiography or radionuclide ventriculography and perfusion imaging, exercise or pharmacologic stress testing more accurately establishes the presence of coronary disease by identifying regions of scarring, inducible ischemia, and/or myocardial viability. Maximal exercise testing with concomitant measurement of oxygen consumption is exceedingly useful in estimating heart failure prognosis. The latter also serves as a guide for an individualized exercise rehabilitation prescription.

Right heart catheterization is most appropriate for patients whose filling pressures and/or cardiac output remain uncertain after physical examination and noninvasive assessment.[35] Additionally, invasive hemodynamic assessment should be considered in patients intolerant of standard therapy or in patients for whom medical therapy has failed to achieve symptomatic relief. Such patients are frequently candidates for inotrope or inodilator therapy.[36]

Noninvasive evaluation of hemodynamic parameters by bioimpedance plethysmography or oscillometric wave analysis may be a surrogate for pulmonary arterial catheterization. However, the accuracy, reproducibility, and clinical use of these diagnostic modalities in heart failure are incompletely defined.

In the absence of sustained or symptomatic ventricular tachycardia, unexplained syncope, or survived sudden death, routine electrophysiologic testing has little diagnostic value, particularly in patients with ischemic

Table 10-6: Prognostic Indicators in Systolic Ventricular Dysfunction*

Patient demographics	Age (older) Gender (? male > female) Race (? African American > white)
Comorbidities	Diabetes Pulmonary hypertension Systemic hypertension Significant renal or hepatic dysfunction Morbid obesity Cachexia Thyroid disease
Symptoms	NYHA classification (IV > III > II > I)
Ejection fraction	Left ventricular ejection fraction (lower) Right ventricular ejection fraction (biventricular > left only)
Left ventricular morphology	Size and volume (larger) Shape (globular) Mass (increased)

* The variables listed to the right of the bolded categories provide prognostic information in chronic heart failure. The presence of a question mark (?) indicates a variable that has been

cardiomyopathy. Endomyocardial biopsy is rarely necessary to establish the etiology of chronic heart failure, but it provides definitive pathologic evidence for several disorders, including primary cardiac amyloidosis, giant cell myocarditis, active cardiac sarcoidosis, and eosinophilic myocarditis.[1,3]

Exercise capacity	VO$_2$ max (lower) Exertional hypotension 6-minute walk distance (<305 m)
Serum sodium	Hyponatremia (<135 mg/dL)
Arrhythmias	Atrial or ventricular (any)
Doppler echo	Restrictive pattern in mitral inflow or pulmonary venous waveform
Neurohormone/ cytokine elevation	Norepinephrine Renin Angiotensin II Aldosterone Natriuretic factors/peptides Endothelin Tumor necrosis factor-α

suggested but not prospectively demonstrated as a prognostic
indicator. The parenthetical information describes the parameter
or directional trend reflecting a more adverse prognosis.

Prognostic Assessment

The evaluation of a patient with chronic heart failure is
incomplete without an initial and periodic assessment of
prognosis that encompasses patient demographics, symptoms, and objective clinical parameters. A summary of
prognostic indicators can be found in Table 10-6.[37] After

Table 10-7: Key Features of Heart Failure Diagnosis and Evaluation

For all patients at risk

- Recognize and modify risk factors for chronic heart failure
- Identify heart failure symptoms when present
- Evaluate for signs of heart failure on physical examination

For patients with symptoms or signs*

- Determine nature and extent of left ventricular dysfunction
- Identify etiology and exacerbating comorbidities
- Evaluate prognosis

* If clinical indecision exists about the diagnosis of heart failure, consider determination of BNP or n-pro BNP level.

institution and titration of standard medical therapy, residual symptoms or persistent adverse prognostic indicators should prompt an assessment for additional therapeutic options and interventions.

Symptoms correlate well with prognosis in systolic LV dysfunction. Despite standard medical therapy, patients with persistent NYHA Class IV symptoms have an annual mortality rate of 40% to 60%, compared with 5% to 10% in NYHA Class I/II patients.[1,3,37] However, NYHA class and objective parameters are not necessarily congruent, which is illustrated by the well-documented lack of correlation between symptoms and LVEF or LVEF and exercise performance in patients with systolic ventricular dysfunction. Each variable examined has independent predictive power.

An LVEF of 30% to 35% reflects a high risk group, particularly among patients with ischemic cardiomyopathy. The greater the degree of decreased contractility (lower ejection fraction), the greater the mortality risk. Right ventricular systolic dysfunction accompanying an impaired LVEF has additive adverse implications. Similarly, the diameter and shape of the left ventricle strongly influence prognosis; increased size and ventricular sphericity correlate with excessive mortality. In patients with systolic LV dysfunction, the finding of impaired diastolic relaxation or a restrictive filling pattern (by Doppler echo) is a powerful predictor of 1-year mortality risk.[26,37]

A severe impairment of objective exercise (functional) capacity, whether measured as maximal exercise capacity (METS or VO_2 max) or submaximal exercise (6-minute walking test distance), is also a strong harbinger of increased annual mortality risk.[37,39] A patient with a VO_2 max <15 mL/kg/min (4 to 5 METS) has a markedly increased 1-year mortality risk (>20%). In certain patients, the exercise performance trend may be more useful, as the prognostic value of the VO_2 max is limited by the absence of well-defined contemporary 'normal' values adjusted for age and gender in many laboratories. Clinical trial data reveal that a patient with systolic LVD who cannot walk more than 300 meters in 6 minutes has a substantially greater annual risk of death than one who can walk 450 meters or more.[39]

Other variables indicating a patient at increased morbidity and mortality risk include the presence and severity of atrial and ventricular arrhythmias, a serum sodium <130 mg/dL, concomitant renal failure, or morbid obesity.[38,40,41] Although not easily or commonly obtained outside of multicenter clinical research trials, neurohormonal markers (norepinephrine, BNP, aldosterone), LV mass, and cardiac histologic findings also yield prognostic information. Table 10-7 lists the key points examined in this chapter.

References

1. Hunt SA, American College of Cardiology; American Heart Association Task Force on Practice Guidelines (Writing Committee to Update the 2001 Guidelines for the Evaluation and Management of Heart Failure): ACC/AHA 2005 guideline update for the diagnosis and management of chronic heart failure in the adult: a report of the American College of Cardiology/American Heart Association Task Force on Practice Guidelines (Writing Committee to Update the 2001 Guidelines for the Evaluation and Management of Heart Failure). *J Am Coll Cardiol* 2005;46:e1-82.

2. Cohn JN, Ferrari R, Sharpe N: Cardiac remodeling—concepts and clinical implications: a consensus paper from an international forum on cardiac remodeling. *J Am Coll Cardiol* 2000;35:569-582.

3. *Heart Failure Society of America*: Executive Summary: HFSA 2006 Comprehensive Heart Failure Practice Guideline. *J Card Fail* 2006;12:10-38. Available at http://www.heartfailureguideline.com.

4. Ghali JK, Kadakia S, Cooper RS, et al: Bedside diagnosis of preserved versus impaired left ventricular systolic function in heart failure. *Am J Cardiol* 1991;67:1002-1006.

5. Chatterjee K: Physical examination in heart failure. In: Hosenpud JD, Greenberg BH, eds. *Congestive Heart Failure. Pathophysiology, Diagnosis and Comprehensive Approach to Management*, 2nd ed. Philadelphia, Lippincott Williams and Wilkins, 2000, pp 615-627.

6. Fuster V, Gersh BJ, Giuliani ER, et al: The natural history of idiopathic dilated cardiomyopathy. *Am J Cardiol* 1981;47:525-531.

7. Gheorghiade M, Bonow RO: Chronic heart failure in the United States: a manifestation of coronary artery disease. *Circulation* 1998;97:282-289.

8. Massie BM, Shah NB: Evolving trends in the epidemiologic factors of heart failure: rationale for preventive strategies and comprehensive disease management. *Am Heart J* 1997;133:703-712.

9. Levy D, Larson MG, Vasan RS, et al: The progression from hypertension to congestive heart failure. *JAMA* 1996;275:1557-1562.

10. Lenihan DJ, Gerson MC, Hoit BD, et al: Mechanisms, diagnosis, and treatment of diastolic heart failure. *Am Heart J* 1995;130:1 53-166.

11. Litwin SE, Grossman W: Diastolic dysfunction as a cause of heart failure. *J Am Coll Cardiol* 1993;22:49A-55A.

12. Topol EJ, Traill TA, Fortuin NJ: Hypertensive hypertrophic cardiomyopathy of the elderly. *N Engl J Med* 1985;312:277-283.

13. Dries DL, Exner DV, Gersh BJ, et al: Racial differences in the outcome of left ventricular dysfunction [published erratum appears in *N Engl J Med* 1999 Jul 22;341:298]. *N Engl J Med* 1999; 340:609-616.

14. Mendes LA, Davidoff R, Cupples LA, et al: Congestive heart failure in patients with coronary artery disease: the gender paradox. *Am Heart J* 1997;134:207-212.

15. Carson P, Ziesche S, Johnson G, et al: Racial differences in response to therapy for heart failure: analysis of the vasodilator-heart failure trials. Vasodilator-Heart Failure Trial Study Group. *J Card Fail* 1999;5:178-187.

16. Aronow WS, Ahn C, Kronzon I: Prognosis of congestive heart failure in elderly patients with normal versus abnormal left ventricular systolic function associated with coronary artery disease. *Am J Cardiol* 1990;66:1257-1259.

17. Chin MH, Goldman L: Gender differences in 1-year survival and quality of life among patients admitted with congestive heart failure. *Med Care* 1998;36:1033-1046.

18. Shindler DM, Kostis JB, Yusuf S, et al: Diabetes mellitus, a predictor of morbidity and mortality in the Studies of Left Ventricular Dysfunction (SOLVD) Trials and Registry. *Am J Cardiol* 1996;77:1017-1020.

19. Hosenpud JD, Jarcho JA: The cardiomyopathies. In: Hosenpud JD, Greenberg BH, eds. *Congestive Heart Failure. Pathophysiology, Diagnosis and Comprehensive Approach to Management*, 2nd ed. Philadelphia, Lippincott Williams and Wilkins, 2000, pp 281-312.

20. Messina E, Giacomello A: Diabetic cardiomyopathy: a "cardiac stem cell disease" involving p66Shc, an attractive novel molecular target for heart failure therapy. *Circ Res* 2006;99:1-2.

21. Hamilton MA, Stevenson LW: Thyroid hormone abnormalities in heart failure: possibilities for therapy. *Thyroid* 1996;6: 527-529.

22. Mielniczuk LM, Williams K, Davis DR, et al: Frequency of peripartum cardiomyopathy. *Am J Cardiol* 2006;97:1765-1768.

23. Fernandez-Sola J, Fatjo F, Sacanella E, et al: Evidence of apoptosis in alcoholic cardiomyopathy. *Hum Pathol* 2006;37:1100-1110.

24. Eisner RM, Husain A, Clark JI: Case report and brief review: IL-2-induced myocarditis. *Cancer Invest* 2004;22:401-404.

25. Brater DC, Harris C, Redfern JS, et al: Renal effects of COX-2-selective inhibitors. *Am J Nephrol* 2001;21:1-15.

26. Pinamonti B, Zecchin M, Di Lenarda A, et al: Persistence of restrictive left ventricular filling pattern in dilated cardiomyopathy: an ominous prognostic sign. *J Am Coll Cardiol* 1997;29:604-612.

27. Cheitlin MD, Alpert JS, Armstrong WF, et al: ACC/AHA guidelines for the clinical application of echocardiography. A report of the American College of Cardiology/American Heart Association Task Force on Practice Guidelines (Committee on Clinical Application of Echocardiography). Developed in collaboration with the American Society of Echocardiography. *Circulation* 1997;95:1686-1744.

28. Ritchie JL, Bateman TM, Bonow RO, et al: Guidelines for clinical use of cardiac radionuclide imaging: a report of the American College of Cardiology/American Heart Association Task Force on Assessment of Diagnostic and Therapeutic Cardiovascular Procedures (Committee on Radionuclide Imaging), developed in collaboration with the American Society of Nuclear Cardiology. *J Am Coll Cardiol* 1995;25:521-547.

29. Nagueh SF: Noninvasive evaluation of hemodynamics by Doppler echocardiography. *Curr Opin Cardiol* 1999;14:217-224.

30. Nishimura RA, Tajik AJ: Evaluation of diastolic filling of left ventricle in health and disease: Doppler echocardiography is the clinician's Rosetta Stone. *J Am Coll Cardiol* 1997;30:8-18.

31. Gallagher MJ, McCullough PA: The emerging role of natriuretic peptides in the diagnosis and treatment of decompensated heart failure. *Curr Heart Fail Rep* 2004;1:129-135.

32. Maisel AS, Krishnaswamy P, Nowak RM, et al: Rapid measurement of B-type natriuretic peptide in the emergency diagnosis of heart failure. *N Engl J Med* 2002;347:161-167.

33. Silver MA, Maisel A, Yancy CW, et al: BNP Consensus Panel 2004: a clinical approach for the diagnostic, prognostic, screening, treatment monitoring, and therapeutic roles of natriuretic peptides in cardiovascular diseases. *Congest Heart Fail* 2004;10(5 suppl 3): 1-30.

34. Morrow DA, de Lemos JA, Blazing MA, et al: Prognostic value of serial B-type natriuretic peptide testing during follow-up of patients with unstable coronary artery disease. *JAMA* 2005;294: 2866-2871.

35. Drazner MH, Hamilton MA, Fonarow G, et al: Relationship between right and left-sided filling pressures in 1000 patients with advanced heart failure. *J Heart Lung Transplant* 1999;18:1126-1132.

36. Connors AF Jr, Speroff T, Dawson NV, et al: The effectiveness of right heart catheterization in the initial care of critically ill patients. SUPPORT Investigators. *JAMA* 1996;276:889-897.

37. Hermann DD, Greenberg BH: Prognostic factors. In: Poole-Wilson PA, et al, eds. *Heart Failure: Scientific Principles and Clinical Practice.* New York, Churchill Livingstone, 1997, pp 439-454.

38. Mortality risk and patterns of practice in 4606 acute care patients with congestive heart failure. The relative importance of age, sex, and medical therapy. Clinical Quality Improvement Network Investigators. *Arch Intern Med* 1996;156:1669-1673.

39. Cahalin LP, Mathier MA, Semigran MJ, et al: The six-minute walk test predicts peak oxygen uptake and survival in patients with advanced heart failure. *Chest* 1996;110:325-332.

40. Davos CH, Doehner W, Rauchhaus M, et al: Obesity and survival in chronic heart failure. *Circulation* 2000;102(suppl I);I-4202.

41. Kjekshus J: Arrhythmias and mortality in congestive heart failure. *Am J Cardiol* 1990;65:42I-48I.

Chapter **11**

Drug Therapy

Those physicians who completed their training before the new millennium have had the opportunity to witness a remarkable turn of events regarding the use of drug therapy in patients with heart failure. Whereas drug therapy for heart failure had previously been considered to be palliative in that it was effective only in relieving symptoms, currently used drugs have been shown beyond a doubt to substantially alter the clinical course of heart failure patients, including prolonging their survival. In this regard, the use of neurohormonal blocking agents such as β-blockers, angiotensin-converting enzyme (ACE) inhibitors, angiotensin-receptor blockers (ARBs), and aldosterone antagonists are now considered to be standard therapy options for treatment of heart failure. An important role for the combination of isosorbide dinitrate and hydralazine has also emerged. Diuretic agents and digoxin have moved from the cornerstones of therapy to a more peripheral position where they are viewed as adjuncts to the other drugs mentioned above. This chapter reviews the rationale for the use of pharmacotherapy in heart failure patients, the relevant clinical trials, and the practical aspects of treatment, such as initiation, up-titration, and management of side effects.

β-Blockers As Effective Therapy

In the patient with impaired left ventricular (LV) systolic function, a variety of local and systemic responses are activated to compensate for a reduction in cardiac output and/or arterial perfusion pressure. Researchers now recognize that although many of these compensatory mechanisms provide important support of cardiac function, they are better suited for short-term protection than for long-term maintenance (eg, the activation of the sympathetic nervous system).[1-3] Catecholamine-mediated increases in heart rate, myocardial contractility, and peripheral vascular tone are ideally suited for acute events, such as dehydration or blood loss, that threaten the viability of the organism. However, when maintained over an extended period in patients with chronic cardiac dysfunction, the effects of catecholamines are now recognized to be highly deleterious. Catecholamines increase vasomotor tone and salt and water retention both directly and by stimulating release of renin activity from the kidney. This increase in plasma renin leads to increases in angiotensin II levels, which promote salt and water retention and peripheral vasoconstriction—effects that lead to worsening heart failure. The resultant increase in wall stress caused by elevated intracardiac pressures and volumes further worsens cardiac function by increasing the load on the failing heart. Down-regulation and desensitization of β-adrenergic receptors in the heart[4] and throughout the body in response to high catecholamine levels compromise the organism's ability to respond to stress by blunting the 'fight or flight' response.

Catecholamines also initiate changes in the structure and function of cells within the heart and throughout the body by stimulating the β_1, β_2, and α_1 receptors, which appears to contribute to the progression of heart failure and its clinical consequences. In particular, adrenergic stimulation of cardiac myocytes stimulates their growth and cardiac hypertrophy is now recognized to have deleterious long-term effects, including decreased survival.

The Emergence of β-Blocker Therapy in Treating Heart Failure Patients

Although the rationale for using β-blockers now seems logical and even intuitive, most of the harmful effects of catecholamines were not clearly defined or recognized 30 years ago when β-blockers were first initiated in heart failure patients. What was widely appreciated at that time was that administration of β-blockers to a patient with LV dysfunction could precipitate worsening heart failure. While this is certainly true, the likelihood of causing a patient's condition to deteriorate can be greatly diminished by using β-blocking drugs in a judicious fashion, including avoiding administration to patients who are acutely decompensated or who have evidence of volume overload. Even more important is the recognition that problems can be successfully avoided in most patients by initiating therapy at a low dose and gradually up-titrating the β-blocker over time. In fact, recent clinical trials with β-blockers have found that these agents are very well tolerated, even in patients with advanced heart failure.

Initial uncontrolled studies in heart failure patients and retrospective analyses of studies that evaluated subgroups of myocardial infarction (MI) survivors with heart failure yielded surprisingly (at the time) positive results for the use of β-blockers in these populations.[5-7] Gradually, these initial encouraging results began to stimulate more widespread interest in the somewhat 'heretical' notion that β-blockers could not only be safely given to heart failure patients, but also might substantially improve patients' clinical course. During the 1980s and early 1990s, several small controlled trials showed that the long-term administration of β-blockers was associated with improvement in the clinical status of heart failure patients.[8-11] Although left ventricular ejection fraction (LVEF) is initially slightly reduced when β-blockers are first administered,[10] there was convincing evidence that maintenance of therapy over several months resulted in a significant (and often dramatic) improvement in cardiac function. Moreover, these patients also experienced improvement in their clinical status, as evidenced by their movement to a lower, more favorable New York Heart Association (NYHA) class.

Results from more ambitious clinical trials assessing the long-term effects of β-blockers played an important role in moving the field forward. However, the initial placebo-controlled trials that included clinically relevant end points, such as the Metoprolol in Dilated Cardiomyopathy (MDC) study[12] and Cardiac Insufficiency Bisoprolol Study I (CIBIS-I),[13] failed to provide convincing evidence of efficacy. Nonetheless, there was a promising reduction, though of borderline statistical significance, in the combined end point of death and need for cardiac transplantation in patients who received metoprolol in the MDC study. Additionally, there was a trend toward a reduction in all-cause mortality in favor of the bisoprolol (Zebeta®)-treated group in CIBIS-I. Although by no means definitive, the results of these relatively small and underpowered studies were highly promising. They also served the important function of drawing attention to the possibility that β-blockers might indeed be useful in treating heart failure patients, and they provided a platform on which the larger studies that eventually proved the 'β-blocker hypothesis' could be constructed. The key studies that provided incontrovertible evidence of the efficacy of β-blockers in treating heart failure patients were US Carvedilol Trial Program[14], CIBIS-II[15], and the MERIT-HF study[16]. All of these studies reported highly significant beneficial effects of β-blockade in heart failure, including an average 35% mortality reduction compared with standard therapy alone. Based on the results of these studies, β-blockers have emerged as one of the 'cornerstones' of treatment for patients with heart failure.

Which β-Blockers
Should Be Used to Treat Heart Failure?

The studies mentioned above strongly support the use of β-blockers in treating heart failure patients. However, the available β-blockers are not a homogeneous group of drugs. A classification of β-blockers based on their pharmacologic properties is shown in Table 11-1. The differences between drugs are based on whether they are selec-

Table 11-1: Classification of β-Blockers

Drug	β_1 Blockade	β_2 Blockade
propranolol (Inderal®)	+	+
atenolol	+	−
metoprolol (Lopressor®, Toprol XL®)	+	−
bisoprolol (Zebeta®)	+	−
carvedilol (Coreg®)	+	+

tive for the β_1-adrenergic receptor, as opposed to providing nonselective blockade of β_1 and β_2 subtypes. Further differentiation is based on whether a particular agent has additional properties, such as α_1-adrenergic blocking properties (that would protect against α_1 stimulation of cardiac cells as well as block α_1-mediated peripheral vasoconstriction) or other vasodilating or antioxidant effects. The three β-blockers proven in mortality trials—bisoprolol (Zebeta®), metoprolol CR/X (Toprol XL®), and carvedilol (Coreg®)—have in common β_1 blockade.

The pharmacokinetics of the drugs may also influence their efficacy in heart failure. The clinical relevance of such differences is shown by the poor initial tolerability of propranolol (Inderal®).[17] This agent depresses contractile function[18] and causes acutely unfavorable hemodynamic effects, including increased systemic vascular resistance, increased pulmonary artery wedge pressure, and reduced cardiac output. Carvedilol is a nonselective β-blocker, but it has additional α_1-blocking effects that pro-

α_1 Blockade	Vasodilation	Other Properties
−	−	−
−	−	−
−	−	−
+	+	Antioxidant

duce vasodilation. This helps unload the heart when the inotropic support, which is mediated through the β_1 and β_2 receptors, is blocked. Consequently, carvedilol is well tolerated, even in patients with advanced heart failure, as was noted in COPERNICUS, a study done in advanced heart failure that will be discussed later in this chapter. Based on these considerations, clinicians can conclude that only β-blockers that have been shown to be effective in large-scale clinical trials (ie, carvedilol, metoprolol CR/XL, and bisoprolol) should be used in treating heart failure patients. Evidence that not all β-blockers should be used in heart failure patients comes from the BEST trial in which bucindolol failed to significantly improve survival in patients with advanced heart failure.[19] This outcome contrasts with the significant improvement in survival in a similar population (in terms of severity of disease) of heart failure patients in the COPERNICUS study who experienced improved survival when carvedilol was added to standard medical therapy.[20]

Results of COMET

The Carvedilol Or Metoprolol European Trial (COMET) recently compared carvedilol and a short-acting formulation of metoprolol tartrate on clinical outcomes in patients with chronic heart failure. This comparison helps provide insight regarding selection of specific β-blocking agents for treating heart failure patients.[21] The multicenter study is a direct head-to-head comparison of carvedilol, a nonspecific β-blocking agent with additional properties, and a short-acting formulation of metoprolol tartrate, a specific β_1-receptor blocker. It compared the effects of these two agents on the clinical course of a group of 3,029 patients with mild to severe heart failure.

The study demonstrated that carvedilol was superior to this short-acting formulation and dose of metoprolol tartrate (Figure 11-1). Overall, patients randomized to carvedilol experienced a 17% reduction in mortality compared to patients randomized to metoprolol tartrate, and carvedilol compared to metoprolol tartrate reduced annual mortality from 10.0% to 8.3%. Carvedilol also prolonged median survival by 1.4 years. Subgroup analysis indicated that the benefits of carvedilol occurred regardless of sex, age, NYHA class, etiology of heart failure, baseline EF, heart rate, systolic blood pressure, or presence of diabetes. The consistency in the results indicates that carvedilol is effective in not just one segment of the population, but across a broad spectrum of heart failure patients. For the composite mortality/morbidity end point, there was a trend toward a more favorable outcome with carvedilol compared to metoprolol tartrate, but it did not achieve statistical significance. Overall, both drugs were well tolerated, and there were no significant differences in adverse events between them.

COMET is the first study to directly compare the effects of two β-blockers in heart failure. These results show that carvedilol provides incremental reductions in heart-failure-related mortality compared with this short-acting formulation and dose of a cardioselective β-blocker.[21] This

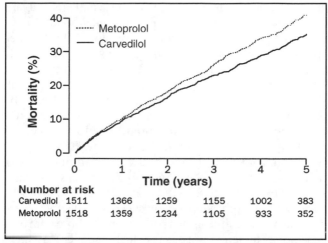

Figure 11-1: Mortality in the Carvedilol Or Metoprolol European Trial (COMET). The hazard ratio was 0.83, with 95% confidence intervals extending from 0.74 to 0.93, P=0.0017. With permission from Poole-Wilson et al, *Lancet* 2003;362:7-13.[21]

reinforces the importance of using a β-blocker proven effective in clinical outcome trials. Specifically, bisoprolol, metoprolol succinate extended-release, or carvedilol have recently been recognized in the revised ACC/AHA guidelines for the treatment of heart failure.[22]

When to Use β-Blockers in Heart Failure Patients

The Guidelines Committee of the Heart Failure Society of America (HFSA) positions β-blocker therapy as standard treatment for heart failure patients.[23] The HFSA recommendations conclude that "β-blockers shown to be effective in clinical trials of patients with heart failure are recommended for patients with LVEF ≤40%."

Now, β-blockers are recommended for treatment of symptomatic patients who have heart failure on the basis of LV systolic dysfunction. Patients should be euvolemic at the time of treatment initiation because patients who are clearly fluid overloaded have a greater likelihood of having an adverse reaction, even when low doses of β-blocker are used. Most heart failure patients show evidence of volume overload, and many have symptoms at rest (eg, Class IV) at some time during the course of their illness. This should not be viewed as an absolute contraindication to β-blocker use, but simply as a sign that such therapy should be temporarily deferred. Initiation of β-blocker therapy should not be attempted until patients are stabilized. β-Blocker therapy should never be used as 'bail-out' therapy for patients who present in an acutely decompensated state, since the benefits manifest only over time. The initial blockade of β-adrenergic support may cause considerable worsening in poorly compensated patients and in those with evidence of volume overload, since such patients may have no margin of reserve to accommodate even a small and temporary decrement in cardiac function.

Initiation of β-blocker therapy does not need to be deferred until after the patient is discharged from the hospital. In most instances low-dose β-blockade can be started after the patient has been stabilized. This approach has been shown to be well tolerated in most instances and it results in a significantly larger number of patients receiving therapy over time.[24] Early treatment also affords protection during the immediate post-hospitalization period which is a time at which patients are known to be at increased risk.

Recent evidence from the COPERNICUS study also suggests that β-blockers (in this case, carvedilol) are well tolerated and effective in reducing mortality in patients with more advanced heart failure.[22] Patients in COPERNICUS had symptoms at rest or with minimal exercise for a period of 2 months or more despite receiving optimal medical management, including, in most cases, an ACE inhibitor or ARB. Patients randomized to carvedilol had a 35% reduction in all-cause mortality, the primary end point in COPERNICUS. In keeping with the COPERNICUS entry criteria, patients with more advanced heart failure who are being considered for β-blocker therapy should be euvolemic at the time of therapy initiation.

Some experts have had success initiating and maintaining β-blockers in patients with even more severe heart failure who require IV inotropic therapy. In these cases, the β-blocker is initiated while the patient is in the hospital and under careful observation for evidence of further compromise of his or her already tenuous state. Since β-agonists, such as dobutamine, compete with the β-blocker for β-receptor occupancy, β-blocker therapy is usually initiated using milrinone, a phosphodiesterase inhibitor, to provide inotropic support. The effects of milrinone are not inhibited by the concomitant administration of a β-blocker, since this drug bypasses the β-receptor and improves contractility by blocking the breakdown of cyclic adenosine monophosphate (cAMP). In our experience, initiation of β-blocker therapy in this population can, in many cases, improve cardiac function to the extent that inotropic therapy can be discontinued over time. However, the use of β-blockers in patients who require inotropic therapy remains investigational, and such therapy should be administered only by heart failure specialists who are experienced in this area.

Use of β-Blockers in Asymptomatic Patients

Little data exist that describe the efficacy of β-blocker therapy in patients with asymptomatic (ie, NYHA Class I) LV dysfunction. However, a strong case can be made for using β-blockers in such patients, based on the fact that early activation of the sympathetic nervous system is involved in the progression of heart failure[4] and on data from limited, but generally promising, studies that incorporated asymptomatic patients. The Australia-New Zealand (ANZ) study evaluated the long-term effects of β-blockers in patients with cardiac dysfunction caused by underlying ischemic disease.[25] Approximately 30% of the population was asymptomatic at the time of randomization to either carvedilol or placebo. For the two primary end points of

Table 11-2: Dose Initiation and Target Dose of β-Blockers

Drug	Initiation Dose	Target Dose
carvedilol	3.125 mg b.i.d.	25 mg b.i.d. (50 mg b.i.d. in patients >85 kg)
bisoprolol	1.25 mg q.d.	10 mg q.d.
metoprolol CR/XL	25 mg q.d. (12.5 mg q.d. in NYHA Class III-IV patients)	200 mg q.d.

the study, carvedilol significantly increased the LVEF but had no significant effect on exercise performance. The results showed that carvedilol was associated with a 26% reduction (P=0.02) in disease progression, a combined end point consisting of mortality, hospitalizations, and sustained requirement for an increase in heart failure medication. There was also evidence that patients treated with carvedilol experienced a reduction in LV volume, a phenomenon termed *reverse remodeling*. Since adverse LV remodeling plays a critical role in the progressive deterioration in cardiac function, such improvements in cardiac structure are believed to be related to the clinical benefits of β-blocker therapy.

How to Use β-Blockers in Heart Failure

As we have seen during the past several years, β-blockers can be safely and easily initiated, up-titrated, and maintained in most heart failure patients. The most important rule of thumb in starting a patient on a β-blocker is to start at a low dose and gradually up-titrate. Table 11-2 gives the starting and target doses for β-blockers that have been shown to be effective in treating heart failure patients in large-scale clinical trials. When a drug is started, patients should be counseled about the possible side effects and given instructions to weigh themselves on a daily basis (a good practice in all heart failure patients). Patients should be urged to contact the clinic if they experience increased shortness of breath, weight gain exceeding 2 pounds over any 2-day period or more than 4 pounds over the course of a 7-day period, symptoms of persistent lightheadedness, or syncope or near syncope.

Side Effects

The main side effects of β-blocker therapy of heart failure are fluid retention, hypotension, and bradycardia. A hierarchical approach to treating these side effects is outlined in Table 11-3.

Patients Who Deteriorate on Therapy

Results from clinical trials have shown that deterioration of cardiac function caused by adding a β-blocker to the medical regimen is much less common than expected. This is related to selection (avoiding patients who are volume overloaded or decompensated) and careful dosing of the drug. When evidence of deterioration is seen, it most often occurs during initiation or up-titration of the drug. If this is the case and the patient does not respond to an increase in the diuretic dose, it is prudent to reduce (at least temporarily) the dose of the β-blocker. Although β-blocker therapy results in substantial improvement in cardiac function, relief of symptoms, and a reduction in hospitalization and emergency department visits, most patients continue to have evidence of LV dysfunction and remain at risk for deterioration. The same well-recognized factors that lead to decompensation of heart failure in patients not on β-blockers are the most common causes of clinical deterioration in patients who are receiving these agents. Thus, consideration should be given to the possibility that clinical decompensation was caused by noncompliance with the medical regimen or diet or by infection, anemia, worsening or comorbid conditions, or other causes.

Table 11-3: Management of the Most Common Side Effects of β-Blocker Therapy in Heart Failure Patients

Side Effect(s)	Strategy
Lightheadedness, hypotension	• Instruct patient to take β-blocker and ACE inhibitor (or other vasodilator) at separate times (usually 2 h apart) • If on carvedilol, take drug with meals to slow absorption • Reduce or discontinue non-ACE inhibitor vasodilators • Reduce diuretic dose in euvolemic, stable patients • Reduce ACE inhibitor dose (temporarily)
Worsening congestive signs/symptoms (eg, increased SOB, orthopnea, PND, ankle swelling)	• Assess patient's compliance with diet/drug therapy and determine if other conditions known to worsen heart failure are present • Increase diuretics • Decrease β-blocker dose if above strategies are not successful
Bradycardia	• Decrease digoxin dose (or calcium-channel blocker) • Reduce β-blocker dose • Consider pacemaker

ACE = angiotensin-converting enzyme
SOB = shortness of breath
PND = paroxysmal nocturnal dyspnea

Patients Presenting
With Profound Decompensation of Heart Failure

Patients who develop profound decompensation of heart failure present a difficult problem, particularly if they require inotropic therapy to stabilize their condition. Although a direct-acting β-agonist, such as dobutamine, may work in such cases, the competition between β-blocker and β-agonist at the level of the cardiac β-receptors tends to make this approach more difficult, and higher doses of the β-agonist than might ordinarily be required are needed. A better approach is to use an agent, such as milrinone, that acts distal to the β-receptor in the adrenergic signaling pathway in stimulating myocardial contractility. In these cases, the β-blocker is continued (or sometimes reduced temporarily until the patient recovers) unless the patient is so profoundly ill that it is essential to provide as much inotropic support as possible. In these instances, β-blockers should be reduced in dose or discontinued.

Patients Who Greatly Improve (or Normalize)
Their Ejection Fraction

Improvement in EF with β-blockers is common, and the usual increase is 5 to 10 EF units or more; normalization of EF may even occur in some patients. There is little reported evidence about the effects of discontinuing β-blockers in this group. When discontinuation was attempted in a small group of 24 patients who improved considerably with β-blockers, evidence of deterioration was documented in two thirds of the group.[26]

Renin-Angiotensin-Aldosterone Blockers

For more than 3 decades, a basic tenet of the pathogenesis of heart failure has been that the renin-angiotensin system (RAS) plays an important role in its development. What is perhaps most interesting (and somewhat unexpected) is that our understanding of the role of the RAS in the development of heart failure has steadily expanded over time, and further insights continue to be revealed. Initially, RAS activation was be-

303

lieved to influence the development and progression of heart failure by hemodynamic effects alone. However, convincing evidence now shows that the RAS promotes cardiac remodeling, a process critical to the progressive worsening in systolic and diastolic function, which ultimately results in heart failure.

There is also more recent evidence demonstrating that the impact of the RAS on the heart may be considerably broader in scope than was initially realized, including the role of the RAS in conditions such as hypertension, left ventricular hypertrophy (LVH), coronary artery atherosclerosis, progressive renal dysfunction, and coronary thrombosis. All of these are related to the development of cardiac dysfunction or manifestations of heart failure. Not surprisingly, drugs that block the RAS have assumed a central role in the management of patients who have overt heart failure or are at risk for developing this condition in the future. Thus, an understanding of the role of the RAS in the pathogenesis of heart failure and the appropriate settings for initiation of treatment are essential to providing optimal therapy.

ACE Inhibitors

The first available agents to block the RAS were the ACE inhibitors, which were initially developed to treat hypertension. Their efficacy in reducing blood pressure and the risk of end-organ damage is now well established. However, the beneficial effects of ACE inhibitors in treating patients with heart failure at virtually all levels of severity, post-MI patients, and patients at increased risk of developing heart failure because of atherosclerotic disease have now been recognized. Interestingly, as indications for the use of ACE inhibitors have grown, uncertainty about the mechanism(s) responsible for their ability to alter the natural history of important cardiovascular diseases has emerged. Much of the debate centers around the issue of the relative importance of the effects of ACE inhibitors in blocking the production of Ang II vs their effects in enhancing the levels of bradykinin.[27,28] Although no definitive answer to this question has emerged, data appear to show that both of these properties of ACE inhibitors may contribute to their beneficial effects.

ACE inhibitors in the prevention of cardiovascular events and heart failure. There is considerable evidence that the RAS plays an important role in the progression of atherosclerotic disease and in the likelihood of future cardiovascular events. The sources of this hypothesis include epidemiologic surveys indicating that hypertensive patients with high levels of plasma renin activity are at increased risk of cardiovascular events (ie, MI) and genetic studies demonstrating that patients with the DD allele of the ACE gene (which would tend to enhance enzymatic activity leading to increased production of angiotensin II) are also at higher risk of MI.[29] Furthermore, post-hoc analysis of the results of the Studies of Left Ventricular Dysfunction (SOLVD) and Survival and Ventricular Enlargement (SAVE) studies suggests that patients randomized to ACE inhibitors experienced a highly significant reduction in the risk of MI and unstable angina.[30,31]

Definitive proof of the value of blocking the RAS in preventing cardiovascular events is now available from the results of the Heart Outcomes Prevention Evaluation (HOPE) study.[32] This trial enrolled 9,297 patients older than 55 years who did not show manifest LV dysfunction. Patients were selected for inclusion if they were at an increased risk for future events based on presence of coronary, peripheral, or cerebrovascular disease or presence of diabetes and at least one other standard cardiovascular risk factor or evidence of microalbuminuria. Patients enrolled in the HOPE study were randomly assigned to receive either the ACE inhibitor ramipril (Altace®) 10 mg/d or placebo in addition to their other medications. The primary end point of the study was a composite of AMI, stroke, and cardiovascular mortality.

Although the results of the HOPE study were unequivocally in favor of ACE inhibitor therapy, the study did not provide information about the mechanism through which the significant reduction in cardiovascular events was achieved. While it was found that blood pressure was reduced with ramipril, the magnitude of the change in this variable with the drug (3/2 mm Hg for systolic/diastolic pressures) does not seem to be a sufficient explanation for the magnitude of the reduction in cardiovascular events. However, even this point has become controversial since limited information obtained from a small group of patients who underwent ambulatory blood pressure monitoring suggested a much greater blood pressure reduction with ramipril. Despite the absence of information defining the mechanism of the protective effects of ACE inhibition with ramipril in these high-risk patients, there is no question about the implications of the HOPE study. The patients included in the trial are similar to those seen in most office and clinic practices, and the results provide persuasive evidence that such high-risk patients will benefit substantially from ACE inhibitor therapy. Thus, in patients who fulfill HOPE entry criteria, an ACE inhibitor is strongly advised unless there is a contraindication to such therapy.

ACE inhibitors post-MI. Several studies have been designed to assess the efficacy of ACE inhibitors post-MI.[31,33-35] These studies mostly enrolled patients who had evidence of substantial LV damage; some patients were asymptomatic, while others had evidence of heart failure at the time of randomization to an ACE inhibitor or placebo. Despite differences in entry criteria and in the drug used, the studies showed remarkable consistency in their results. All of these trials demonstrated significant reductions in all-cause mortality with ACE inhibitor therapy compared to standard therapy. Overall, the reduction in mortality was 20% to 25% with ACE inhibitor therapy.

In SAVE, patients with an ejection fraction (EF) <0.40 after MI were randomized to captopril (Capoten®) 50 mg t.i.d. or placebo in addition to their other medications.[31] Captopril therapy was associated with a 19% reduction in all-cause mortality (P=0.019), the primary end point of the study. Cardiovascular mortality was reduced by 21%, and recurrent MI was reduced by 25%. The development of heart failure was designated as a secondary end point of the SAVE study, and overall, there was a significant 37% RR (P=0.032) associated with captopril treatment (Figure 11-2). Another example is the Acute Infarction Ramipril Efficiency (AIRE) study.[36] In this trial, patients with clinical evidence of heart failure post-MI were randomized to either ramipril or placebo. The results of the AIRE study showed that ACE inhibitor therapy reduced all-cause mortality by 27% (P=0.002) and the combined end point of death, severe or resistant congestive heart failure (CHF), reinfarction, and stroke by 19% (P=0.008).

ACE inhibitors in patients with asymptomatic LV dysfunction. The prevention arm of SOLVD studied the effects of ACE inhibition in patients with asymptomatic LV dysfunction (ie, LVEF <0.35).[37] Although most patients (more than 80% in the enalapril [Vasotec®] and placebo groups) had underlying coronary artery disease as the cause of their LV dysfunction, entry into the study was precluded for at least 6 months post-MI. Thus, the SOLVD prevention arm population was distinctly different from the patients included in studies evaluating ACE inhibition in the immediate post-MI period. Additionally, a substantial number of patients with a nonischemic etiology of heart failure were included in the study. The 4,228 patients included in the prevention arm of SOLVD were assigned to receive either enalapril 10 mg b.i.d. or placebo in addition to their other medications. Although there was an 8% reduction in the primary end point of all-cause mortality, the results did not achieve statistical significance. However, after an average of 3 years' follow-up, death or hospitalization be-

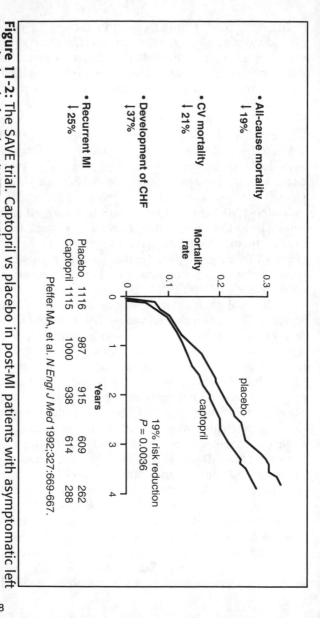

Figure 11-2: The SAVE trial. Captopril vs placebo in post-MI patients with asymptomatic left ventricular dysfunction (LVEF ≤0.40).

- All-cause mortality
  ↓ 19%
- CV mortality
  ↓ 21%
- Development of CHF
  ↓ 37%
- Recurrent MI
  ↓ 25%

Mortality rate

Placebo	1116	987	915	609	262
Captopril	1115	1000	938	614	288

Years

placebo

captopril

19% risk reduction
P = 0.0036

Pfeffer MA, et al. *N Engl J Med* 1992;327:669-667.

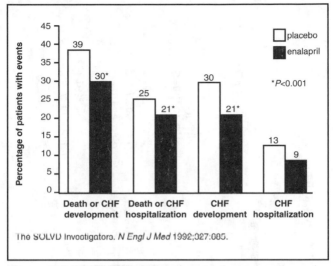

The SOLVD Investigators. N Engl J Med 1992;327:685.

Figure 11-3: SOLVD prevention trial. Enalapril vs placebo in 4,228 patients with asymptomatic left ventricular dysfunction (LVEF ≤35%).

cause of heart failure was reduced by 20%, death or development of heart failure was reduced by 29%, development of heart failure was reduced by 37%, and heart failure hospitalizations were reduced by 44% (all *P*<0.001), as shown in Figure 11-3.

ACE inhibitors in patients with symptomatic LV dysfunction. The treatment arm of SOLVD assessed the effects of ACE inhibitors in patients with mild to moderate symptoms of heart failure associated with a reduced LVEF.[38] The study included 2,579 patients with heart failure from either ischemic or nonischemic causes. As in the prevention arm, patients were randomly assigned to receive either enalapril 10 mg b.i.d. or placebo in addition to their other heart failure medications, such as digoxin, diuretics (eg, furosemide [Lasix®]), and non-ACE inhibitor vasodilators.

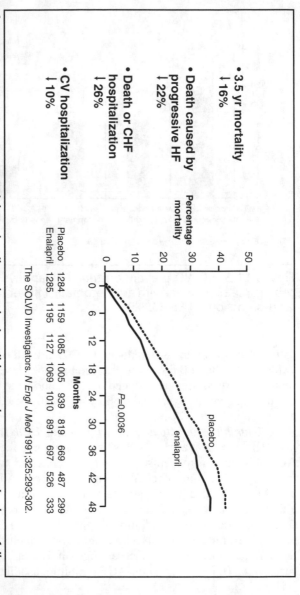

- **3.5 yr mortality**
  ↓ 16%
- **Death caused by progressive HF**
  ↓ 22%
- **Death or CHF hospitalization**
  ↓ 26%
- **CV hospitalization**
  ↓ 10%

Placebo	1284	1159	1085	1005	939	819	669	487	299
Enalapril	1285	1195	1127	1069	1010	891	697	526	333

The SOLVD Investigators. *N Engl J Med* 1991;325:293-302.

P=0.0036

Figure 11-4: SOLVD treatment trial. Enalapril vs placebo in mild to moderate congestive heart failure (CHF) with LVEF ≤0.35.

After an average 3.5-year follow-up, there was a highly significant 16% reduction ($P=0.0036$) in all-cause mortality, the primary end point of the study (Figure 11-4). Cardiovascular hospitalizations were reduced by 10%, death caused by progressive heart failure was reduced by 22%, and death or heart failure hospitalizations were reduced by 26% ($P<0.00001$).

Effects of ACE inhibitors on LV remodeling in the SOLVD study. As part of SOLVD, a group of 300 representative patients underwent serial echo-Doppler evaluation over the course of the first 12 months after randomization to ACE inhibitor or placebo.[39] The study included prevention- and treatment-arm patients, and the results were pooled together when analysis showed no significant interaction between the effects of therapy and the patient arm of the study. The results of the changes in cardiac structure with ACE inhibitor therapy are summarized in Table 11-4. They show that at baseline, LV volumes and mass in this subgroup of SOLVD patients were considerably elevated compared with a control population, indicating that the study patients had already undergone substantial amounts of LV remodeling. Over the 12-month follow-up period, significant increases in LV volume and mass occurred in the patients randomized to placebo. These results show that cardiac remodeling in patients with LV dysfunction is a progressive process and that the adverse changes in cardiac structure continue to develop over an extended period. Patients treated with enalapril, however, demonstrated inhibition of further increase in LV volume or mass. Over the course of the study, the differences in the changes in LV structure between the placebo- and enalapril-treated patients were significant. These results show the protective effect of ACE inhibition on progressive LV remodeling. They suggest that the beneficial effects of enalapril on the natural history of patients with LV dysfunction seen in the SOLVD trials are partly the result of enalapril's ability to prevent further heart remodeling from occurring.

311

Table 11-4: Effects of Enalapril on Cardiac Remodeling in SOLVD

Variable	Treatment	Baseline
EDV (mL)	P	200 ± 42
	E	196 ± 41
	C	131 ± 30
ESV (mL)	P	148 ± 38
	E	146 ± 38
	C	64 ± 25
LV mass (g)	P	280 ± 100
	E	265 ± 82
	C	133 ± 45

EDV = end-diastolic volume; ESV = end-systolic volume; LV = left ventricular; P = placebo; E = enalapril; C = control; B = baseline.

ACE inhibitors in patients with advanced LV dysfunction. Patients enrolled in the Cooperative North Scandinavian Enalapril Survival Study (CONSENSUS) had New York Heart Association (NYHA) Class IV symptoms of heart failure with LV systolic dysfunction. The 253 patients enrolled in this trial were randomly assigned to receive either enalapril or placebo in addition to their standard heart failure therapy. Confirmation of heart failure severity in the CONSENSUS population came from the observation that mortality in the placebo-treated patients was approximately 50% at 6 months.[40] The addition of an ACE inhibitor had a profound influence on the clinical course of these patients. Enalapril reduced 6-month mortality by 40% (*P*=0.002) and 1-year mortality by 31% (*P*=0.001). Death

P value 12 Months	P value (B vs 12M)	(P vs E)
210 ± 46	0.003	0.025
197 ± 39	0.852	
156 ± 42	0.014	0.019
145 ± 38	0.594	
297 ± 100	0.178	<0.001
255 ± 82	0.280	

caused by progressive heart failure was reduced by 50% (*P*=0.001). Additionally, evidence showed that enalapril reduced NYHA class, heart size, and medication use in the CONSENSUS study population.

Recommendations for the use of ACE inhibitors in the prevention and treatment of heart failure. All of the trials described were double-blinded, placebo-controlled, and adequately sized to assess morbidity and mortality end points. Based on these results, recommendations regarding the use of ACE inhibitors can be offered (Table 11-5). Basically, ACE inhibitors should be used in a broad spectrum of patients who either have heart failure or are at risk for developing it. Their value is more extensive than was initially thought when the drugs were first approved to treat

Table 11-5: Recommendations for the Use of ACE Inhibitors to Prevent and/or Treat Heart Failure

- Post-MI patients, regardless of EF
- Patients with diabetes and one of the following:
  - hypertension
  - elevated total cholesterol
  - low HDL cholesterol
  - cigarette smoking
  - microalbuminuria
- NYHA Class II, III, IV heart failure
- Asymptomatic LV dysfunction with an EF ≤0.40

ACE = angiotensin-converting enzyme
EF = ejection fraction
MI = myocardial infarction
HDL = high-density lipoprotein
NYHA = New York Heart Association
LV = left ventricular

patients with symptomatic heart failure. Now there is compelling evidence that ACE inhibitor use should extend all the way from patients who are at risk for cardiovascular events to those who have severe NYHA Class IV symptoms of heart failure. This includes MI survivors and patients with LV dysfunction, regardless of symptomatic state.

ACE inhibitors are usually initiated at a low dose and then up-titrated to the desired dose over a few days to weeks. The initial and optimal doses of approved ACE inhibitors are shown in Table 11-6. Before initiation of therapy, patients should have blood drawn for measurement of electrolytes and renal function. Patients with hyperkalemia should not begin taking the ACE inhibitor until

Table 11-6: ACE Inhibitors Approved for Treatment of Heart Failure and LV Dysfunction

| Agent | Indication | | Dose |
	HF	LV Dysfunction	
captopril (Capoten®)	√	√ (post-MI)	6.25 mg-50 mg t.i.d.
enalapril (Vasotec®)	√	√ (asymptomatic)	2.5 mg-10 mg b.i.d.
fosinopril (Monopril®)	√	NA	20 mg-40 mg q.d.
lisinopril (Prinivil®, Zestril®)	√	√ (post-MI)	5 mg-20 mg q.d.
quinapril (Accupril®)	√	NA	10 mg-20 mg b.i.d.
ramipril (Altace®)	√	√ (post-MI)	2.5-5 mg b.i.d.
trandolapril (Mavik®)	√	√ (post-MI)	1 mg-4 mg q.d.

ACE = angiotensin-converting enzyme
LV = left ventricular
HF = heart failure
MI = myocardial infarction

this condition has been satisfactorily treated and it is clear that the cause of the high potassium levels has been corrected. Abnormal renal function is a relative contraindication to the use of ACE inhibitors because the effects of these drugs on blood pressure and intrarenal hemodynamics are likely to result in a worsening of this condition. However, most heart failure experts will initiate therapy with ACE inhibitors in patients with serum creatinine levels <2.5 to 3.0 mg/dL. Although a further rise in the creatinine level is likely to occur, it is important to recognize that this does not indicate irreversible renal damage, but rather altered kidney function that can usually be reversed with discontinuation of the ACE inhibitor.

The decision to stop an ACE inhibitor, maintain the drug at a less-than-optimal dose, or reduce the dose should be based on whether there is evidence of tissue hypoperfusion. This is usually manifested by either lightheadedness and dizziness (caused by cerebral hypoperfusion) or by more serious evidence of renal dysfunction than outlined earlier. This approach allows appropriate up-titration of the drug in patients who appear to have borderline blood pressures and provides guidelines for restraint in dosing patients who cannot tolerate therapy despite 'normal' blood pressure.

Angioedema is a serious side effect of ACE inhibitor therapy that can be life-threatening in severe cases. Its prevalence is estimated to be <1%, but it is more common in African Americans. Angioedema is an indication to permanently discontinue ACE inhibitor therapy. Cough is a troublesome side effect of the ACE inhibitors that occurs in approximately 5% to 10% of patients. However, its incidence may be higher in selected populations. It is important to distinguish ACE inhibitor-mediated cough from cough caused by other reasons in the heart failure population. Continuation of cough after other causes have been excluded may be a reason to discontinue therapy in some patients with severe symptoms.

Angiotensin-receptor Blockers in the Treatment of Heart Failure

Angiotensin-receptor blockers (ARBs) are a more contemporary class of drugs used to block the RAS. They are pharmacologically distinct from ACE inhibitors and offer an alternative means for blocking the effects of Ang II rather than its synthesis.[41,42] ARBs, in contrast to ACE inhibitors, block the interaction between Ang II and the AT_1 receptor regardless of the source of the peptide. Thus, it is irrelevant whether Ang II was generated by ACE or through an alternative pathway that uses enzymes such as chymase. However, ACE inhibitors have additional effects that are potentially important in the pathogenesis of cardiovascular disease; they also block the breakdown of bradykinin, a peptide with effects that may be relevant to the pathogenesis of a variety of cardiovascular diseases.[43]

There is also evidence that the ARBs may affect alternative pathways of the RAS in ways that could be important in the treatment of cardiovascular diseases. Recently, a homologue of ACE, termed ACE2, has been identified.[44] This enzyme prefers Ang II as its substrate and acts to cleave the terminal acid from the octapeptide to form Ang-(1-7), a heptapeptide that appears to possess vasodilatory and antigrowth effects. Thus, the ACE2/Ang-(1-7) pathway may be cardioprotective, acting to reduce the production of Ang II while it increases production of a counter-regulatory peptide. In the rat model of MI, the administration of an ARB increased ACE2 expression in the heart and increased plasma concentrations of Ang-(1-7).[45]

ARB therapy to prevent heart failure. The use of ARB therapy to prevent progression of disease and as a way to reduce risk has been assessed in patients with type II diabetes, proteinuria, and elevated serum creatinine levels in the Reduction of End Points in Non-Insulin Dependent Diabetes Mellitus with the Angiotensin II Antagonist Losartan (RENAAL) trial. Of the 1,513 patients enrolled in RENAAL, 92% had hypertension in addition to diabetes. Although these patients were receiving a variety of drugs to treat their hypertension, the use of an ACE inhibitor or an ARB at the time of randomization was not allowed. Patients who met the entry criteria were randomized to receive placebo or losartan (Cozaar®) 50 to 100 mg q.d. in addition to their other medications. Over a mean follow-up period of 3.4 years, fewer patients discontin-

Table 11-7: Results of RENAAL

- Primary composite end point (eg, doubling of serum creatinine; ESRD; death) was reduced 16% (P=0.024) with losartan

- Losartan reduced the components of the primary end point as follows:
  - 28% reduction in ESRD (P=0.002)
  - 25% reduction in doubling serum creatinine (P=0.006)
  - no significant mortality effect
  - 20% reduction in death or ESRD (P=0.010)

- Addition of losartan affected other end points:
  - 35% reduction in proteinuria (P=0.000)
  - 32% reduction in HF hospitalization (P=0.005)

RENAAL = Reduction of End Points in Non-Insulin-Dependent Diabetes Mellitus with the Angiotensin II Antagonist Losartan
ESRD = end-stage renal disease
HF = heart failure

ued losartan than placebo (17% vs 22%). The primary end point of this study was a composite of end-stage renal disease (ESRD), a two-fold increase in serum creatinine level, or death. The results of RENAAL are summarized in Table 11-7. At the time that the study was stopped, there was a 16% reduction in the primary composite end point in the losartan-treated patients.

This effect of losartan was statistically significant and was caused predominantly by the protective effects of losartan on renal function, as evidenced by the 28% reduction in ESRD and the 25% reduction in the likelihood of increased creatinine levels. Thus, the addition of losartan to this high-risk, mostly diabetic, hypertensive population reduced the future likelihood of deterioration in renal function. Based on the presence of potent cardiovascular risk factors, clinicians would anticipate that the RENAAL population would be at relatively high risk for developing heart failure. The addition of losartan, however, reduced this risk considerably, as evidenced by the 32% reduction in heart failure hospitalizations ($P=0.005$) compared to the placebo group.

ARBs as alternatives to ACE inhibitors in the treatment of heart failure. The possibility that treatment with an ARB might have more favorable effects on survival in heart failure patients was assessed in the Evaluation of Losartan in the Elderly II (ELITE II) study.[46] There was great enthusiasm for this possibility based on the results of the ELITE I study, which had demonstrated a nearly 50% lower mortality with losartan compared to captopril in elderly ACE inhibitor-naive patients.[47] Interestingly, ELITE I had not been designed to assess mortality as an end point of the study. The primary end point of ELITE I was the effect of an ARB vs an ACE inhibitor on renal function in a heart failure population. The results of ELITE I demonstrated conclusively that there was essentially no significant difference in the likelihood of a clinically important rise in serum creatinine between the treatments. Thus, the ELITE I study demonstrated that both ACEs and ARBs were well tolerated by the kidneys. The ELITE II study was then constructed to test the hypothesis that losartan 50 mg q.d. would reduce mortality by 20% when compared to a control population that was treated with the ACE inhibitor captopril 50 mg t.i.d. Patients enrolled in ELITE II were older than 54 years and were ACE inhibitor naive. They were required to have symptomatic heart failure (ie, NYHA Class II-IV) and an LVEF <0.40. The results of the study did not support the hypothesis that losartan had a more favorable effect on mortality than captopril. The life table curves for the two treatment regimens for all-cause mortality, the primary end point of the study, were not significantly different. For secondary end points, such as quality of life and NYHA class, there were significant improvements with either drug and no significant differences in the response between them. Losartan, however, was better tolerated than captopril. Withdrawals and drug discontinuation occurred because of adverse advents with losartan and captopril such as cough and worsening CHF.

Other studies evaluating the effects of ARBs as an alternative to ACE inhibitors have provided important insights about the value of ARBs in treating heart failure. The Valsartan in Heart Failure Trial (Val-HeFT) was designed primarily to assess the effects of the addition of an ARB to ACE inhibitor therapy; the results are examined in the next section of this chapter. A subgroup of the Val-HeFT patients (n=366, or 7.3% of the study population) was not, however, taking an ACE inhibitor, and the results of treatment in these patients allowed the investigators to assess the effects of ARB therapy in heart failure patients.[48] The results depicted in Figure 11-5 show that in this subgroup, the patients who received valsartan (Diovan®) experienced a 44% reduction in the combined mortality/morbidity end point ($P<0.001$).

Even more convincing evidence of the efficacy of ARBs in the treatment of heart failure is from the Candesartan in Heart Failure Assessment of Reduction in Mortality and morbidity Alternative Trial (CHARM-Alternative).[49] In this study, the effects of candesartan (Atacand®, n=1,013) were compared to placebo (n=1,015) in heart failure patients who were intolerant of ACE inhibitors but were receiving other standard therapies for the treatment of heart failure. Doses of candesartan were started at 4 mg once daily and gradually increased to a target dose of 32 mg once daily. Overall, there was a robust 23% risk reduction ($P<0.0004$) in

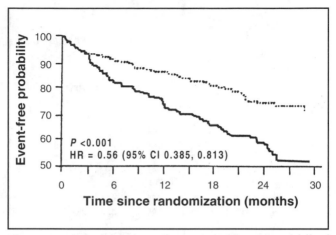

Figure 11-5: Valsartan reduces combined morbidity/ mortality in the subgroup (n = 366) of patients not receiving ACE inhibitor background therapy. The figure depicts Kaplan-Meier curves for patients in valsartan (dotted) and placebo (solid) groups of the Val-HeFT study. HR = hazard ratio. From Maggioni et al.[48]

the combined end point of cardiovascular death or heart failure hospitalization (Figure 11-6). As shown in Figure 11-7, this effect was due to a reduction in both components of the composite end point.

Effects of combined ACE inhibitor and ARB therapy. The Val-HeFT study was designed to determine if the combination of an ARB and an ACE inhibitor significantly improved the natural history of patients with heart failure compared to the effects of ACE inhibitor therapy alone. Val-HeFT included patients with evidence of LV dysfunction and symptomatic heart failure despite standard therapy, including an ACE inhibitor. Patients were randomly assigned to either placebo or valsartan started at 40 mg b.i.d. and titrated to 160 mg b.i.d. The two primary end points of the trial were all-cause mortality and

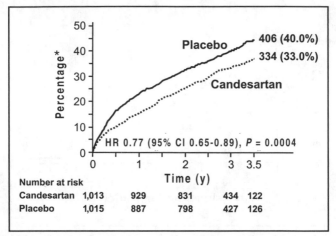

Figure 11-6: Primary end-point results from the CHARM-Alternative study. Patients treated with candesartan experienced a highly significant 23% reduction in risk for the combined end points of cardiovascular deaths or heart failure hospitalizations. HR = hazard ratio. *Percentage of patients experiencing combined end point. From Granger et al.[49]

combined mortality and morbidity. No significant benefit in mortality reduction was seen with combined therapy compared to ACE inhibitor treatment alone. However, the combined mortality and morbidity end point was reduced by 13.3% (P=0.009) by the addition of valsartan to the ACE inhibitor. This reduction was largely caused by a highly significant 27.5% reduction in heart failure hospitalization with combined ARB/ACE inhibitor therapy.

The CHARM-Added study evaluated the effects of candesartan (n=1,276) or placebo (n=1,272) on the treatment regimen of symptomatic heart failure patients with ejection fraction ≤0.40 who were already receiving an ACE inhibitor.[50] As with the CHARM-Alternative study,

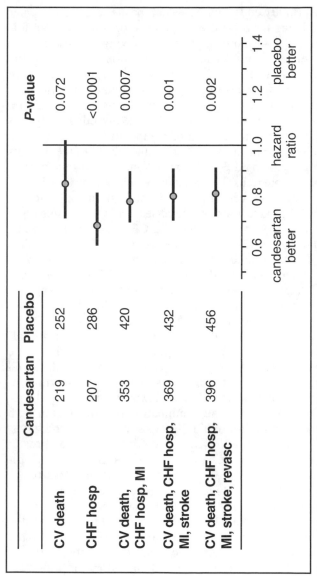

Figure 11-7: Results of the CHARM-Alternative study. From Granger et al.[49]

the primary end point was a composite of cardiovascular death and heart failure hospitalization. At a median follow-up of 41 months, patients receiving candesartan experienced a significant 15% reduction ($P=0.01$) in the composite end point. Moreover, candesartan reduced each of the components of the primary outcome significantly, as well as the total number of admissions for heart failure. An important analysis of the CHARM-Added study was related to the interaction of combination treatment with β-blockers and an ARB. In this study, 55% of the patients were receiving a β-blocker, and analysis of this interaction was predefined in the study design. The results showed that patients receiving an ACE inhibitor and a β-blocker as background therapy did at least as well as those patients who were receiving the ACE inhibitor alone when candesartan was added to the regimen.

The beneficial effects of adding an ARB to standard treatment that already included an ACE inhibitor, demonstrated in the CHARM-Added study, is consistent with earlier results of the Randomized Evaluation of Strategies for Left Ventricular Dysfunction (RESOLVD) pilot study.[51] This study was designed to provide information about the effects of candesartan, enalapril, or the combination of agents on a variety of heart failure end points, as well as these agents in combination with a β-blocker (metoprolol succinate–extended release). The results showed that the combination of candesartan with an ACE inhibitor and a β-blocker resulted in the greatest increase in LV ejection fraction as well as greater attenuation of increases in LV systolic and diastolic volumes compared to treatment with either candesartan or enalapril alone. Because therapy, which favorably affects the remodeling process, usually has beneficial effects on the clinical course of heart failure patients, the results of RESOLVD predicted the outcomes of the CHARM-Added study, including the beneficial effects of adding candesartan to an ACE inhibitor plus β-blocker.

We now recognize that approximately half of the patients admitted to hospital with heart failure have preserved ejection fraction. The CHARM-Preserved study was the first to target heart failure patients with preserved ejection fraction.[52] In this trial, patients with symptoms of heart failure and an LV ejection fraction >0.40 were assigned to receive either candesartan (n=1,514) or placebo (n=1,509) in addition to their current treatment. After a median follow-up of 36.6 months, candesartan-treated patients experienced an 11% reduction (P=0.118) in risk for the composite end point of cardiovascular death or heart failure hospitalization. Fewer patients in the candesartan group than in the placebo group were hospitalized for heart failure (P=0.017), and there was a reduction in the overall number of hospitalizations in these patients. An ongoing study (I-PRESERVE) evaluating the effects of an ARB in treating patients with heart failure and preserved ejection fraction should provide needed additional information about this approach.

Role of ARBs in preventing and treating heart failure. Until recently, information about the role of ARBs in treating patients with heart failure has been limited, in large part because the ARBs became available only after ACE inhibitors had already become a standard of therapy for this condition. That situation has now been largely corrected by the publication of results from the ELITE, Val-HeFT, and CHARM trials, providing convincing evidence that ARBs are an effective therapy for treating patients with heart failure. Based primarily on the results of the CHARM-Alternative study, the FDA has recently approved the use of candesartan for the treatment of heart failure (NYHA class II-IV and ejection fraction ≤40%) to reduce the risk of death from cardiovascular causes and reduce hospitalizations for heart failure. When candesartan is selected as an alternative to an ACE inhibitor, it should be started at a dose of 4 mg and then gradually titrated to a target dose of 32 mg.

Inhibition of Aldosterone in Heart Failure
Aldosterone 'escape'

Patients with heart failure may have high levels of circulating aldosterone despite treatment with an ACE inhibitor or an ARB, a condition referred to as *aldosterone escape*.[53] Aldosterone release from the adrenal gland is influenced by factors other than Ang II. Aldosterone is known to have a variety of effects throughout the body. In the kidney, it promotes salt and water retention, as well as loss of potassium and magnesium. Aldosterone has also been associated with sympathetic stimulation and parasympathetic inhibition, baroreceptor dysfunction, vascular damage, and impaired arterial compliance. In addition, a considerable body of evidence suggests that aldosterone is an important factor in the development of cardiac fibrosis.[54,55] The deposition of fibrous tissue is increased in the failing heart, and the quantity and structure of the extracellular matrix (ECM) component of the myocardium are important determinants of systolic and diastolic function. Thus, it appears that aldosterone may play an important role in the pathogenesis of the deleterious heart remodeling that has been implicated in the progression of cardiac dysfunction.

The role of aldosterone blockade in patients with severe heart failure was assessed in the Randomized Aldactone Evaluation Study (RALES) in which 1,663 patients with severe heart failure due to systolic dysfunction were already being treated with an ACE inhibitor were randomized to receive either spironolactone 25 mg or placebo daily in addition to their standard therapy. At 24 months after randomization, there was a 30% reduction in mortality risk (95% confidence intervals 0.60 to 0.83; p<0.001) in the spironolactone group. Hospitalizations for worsening heart failure were also significantly reduced. Severe hyperkalemia was minimal in both groups but gynecomastia or breast pain was more common in men receiving spironolactone (10%) than placebo (1%).

The use of an aldosterone blocker has been further studied in patients with post-MI left ventricular dysfunction and heart failure in the EPHESUS trial. In this study of 3,313 patients, the addition of eplerenone titrated to 50 mg daily to standard therapy which included both an ACE inhibitor and a β-blocker in the vast majority of patients was associated with a 15% mortality risk reduction (95% confidence intervals 0.75 to 0.96; p=0.008). A small increase in serious hyperkalemia was offset by a significant reduction in the risk of hypokalemia.

Recommendations for the use of aldosterone blockers in treating heart failure patients

Based on the results of RALES, an aldosterone blocker is recommended in patients with advanced heart failure. The results of EPHESUS demonstrate the efficacy of eplerenone (Inspra®) in the post-MI population with LV dysfunction and evidence of heart failure. In EPHESUS, beneficial effects of eplerenone were additive to those of other neurohormonal blocking agents. Thus, the addition of an aldosterone receptor blocker to therapy in such patients is now also indicated. However, the implication of the results of these studies, which examined the use of aldosterone blockade in two distinct patient groups, is that this therapeutic approach may be of value across the spectrum of patients with heart failure caused by LV systolic dysfunction. It is our practice to consider the use of an aldosterone receptor blocking agent in almost all of our patients with heart failure from systolic dysfunction, regardless of whether heart failure is from a recent MI and regardless of the NYHA functional class.

Aldosterone receptor blockers should be added to other agents that have been demonstrated to be of value in treating heart failure. They are used in addition to, not in place of, ACE inhibitors and β-blockers. Contraindications to the use of aldosterone receptor blockers include baseline serum potassium levels >5.0 mEq/L and serum creatinine levels >2.5 mg/dL. For patients receiving potassium supplementation, the dose is usually reduced when an aldosterone receptor blocker is initiated. Reduction of the dose by a third or by half is a reasonable place to begin, but the effect of the drug (even in patients not receiving supplemental potassium) is unpredictable; therefore, potassium blood levels should be measured regularly.

Digitalis, Diuretics, and Vasodilator Therapy

This section reviews the use of adjunctive agents (digitalis, diuretics) and other alternative vasodilator drugs.

Digoxin

Clinical Trial Indications

Despite more than 2 centuries of use and contemporary outcomes data, digitalis use in chronic heart failure remains controversial and is an infrequently prescribed therapy for heart failure in Europe. Sufficient data supporting digoxin (Lanoxin®) use for symptomatic improvement, including quality of life and exercise duration, resulted in the US Food and Drug Administration's approval for its use in mild to moderate heart failure. In addition, the American College of Cardiology/American Heart Association[22] and the Heart Failure Society of America clinical guidelines[23] recommend digoxin use for symptomatic heart failure patients in the absence of specific contraindications (Table 11-8). The data used for these decisions included the Digitalis Investigation Group (DIG) mortality trial[56] sponsored by the National Institutes of Health (NIH), along with retrospective analyses from the Prospective Randomized Study of Ventricular Failure and the Efficacy of Digoxin (PROVED)[57] and the Randomized Assessment of the Effect of Digoxin on Inhibitors of the Angiotensin-Converting Enzyme (RADIANCE) trial databases.[58]

The DIG trial was a randomized, double-blind, placebo-controlled mortality trial enrolling nearly 7,800 heart failure patients on background ACE inhibitor and diuretic therapy.[56] Only a small proportion of patients were receiving a β-blocker at study entry, based on trial data available

Table 11-8: Guidelines for Digoxin Use

- Indicated in NYHA Class II-IV heart failure patients on ACE inhibitors, β-blockers, and diuretics.

- No loading dose necessary in sinus rhythm.

- Dose is 0.125 to 0.250 mg/d depending on age, renal function, and concomitant medications.

- Trough serum concentration 0.8 to 1.2 ng/mL.

ACE = Angiotensin-converting enzyme
NYHA = New York Heart Association

at the time the study was conducted. Most patients (6,800) had heart failure caused by systolic LVD with an ejection fraction (EF) ≤45%. Overall, digitalis administration had a neutral effect on the primary outcome variable of total mortality (35%) after an average follow-up period of approximately 3 years (relative risk ratio [RR] 0.99, P=0.8). Cardiovascular mortality (30%) was also similar in the two groups. Thus, digitalis represents the only available oral agent with mild, positively inotropic activity that does not adversely affect mortality in heart failure populations.

In the DIG trial, digoxin administration had a beneficial effect on the clinical outcome of heart failure patients for the combined secondary trial end point of hospitalization or need for increased heart failure medication (increased diuretic or ACE inhibitor dose or added therapies). Overall, significantly fewer patients on digoxin (26.8%) than placebo (34.7%) were hospitalized for worsening heart failure (RR 0.72 [95% CI 0.66 to 0.79], P<0.001). Further, in a prespecified subgroup analysis of patients with severe heart failure (EF <0.25), a 16% reduction in all-cause mortality or hospitalization was noted for patients receiving digoxin (95% CI 0.07 to 0.24). More notably, heart failure death or hospitalization was reduced by 39% for those patients with severe heart failure who were randomized to digoxin therapy vs placebo (95% CI 0.29 to 0.47). Digoxin is generally administered to patients with systolic LVD.

Additional evidence showing that digoxin use has additive benefits to ACE inhibitor therapy derives from a contemporary analysis of the combined PROVED and RADIANCE trial databases.[57,58] When digitalis administration was continued along with an ACE inhibitor and diuretic background therapy, only 4.7% of patients were hospitalized for worsening heart failure. This was significantly less than the 25% of patients on an ACE inhibitor and diuretic combination hospitalized after digoxin withdrawal (P=0.001). Hospitalization occurred in 39% of patients withdrawn from digitalis therapy and maintained on diuretic monotherapy (P<0.001) and in 19% of those continued on digoxin and diuretics but without an ACE inhibitor (P=0.009).

Mechanism of Action

Aside from digoxin's electrophysiologic effects, the traditional perception of digoxin's effect on the cardiovascular system in heart failure is that it is a mild positive inotropic agent. This perception is based on the long-known ability of digoxin to inhibit myocardial membrane sodium-potassium adenosine triphosphatase (ATPase) activity. The resultant increase in intracellular calcium concentration through sodium-calcium exchange increases myocardial contractility. Globally, ventricular function (Frank-Starling) curves shift upward and leftward, reflecting increased cardiac work at the same filling pressure. This corresponds to an approximately 5% global increase in LVEF.

Digoxin has also been shown to possess sympathoinhibitory neurohormonal modulating effects, which are probably responsible for its beneficial effects in heart failure.[59,60]

Clinical Prescription and Monitoring

Although several digitalis glycoside formulations exist, the most widely prescribed form is digoxin. Compounds in gel form have 90% to 100% bioavailability, although drugs that increase gastrointestinal motility can reduce absorption, as do binding resins, such as cholestyramine (Questran®) and some antacids. There is no evidence that tachyphylaxis occurs with chronic administration.

For the treatment of chronic heart failure in sinus rhythm, a loading dose is unnecessary. The recommended dose ranges from 0.125 to 0.250 mg/d, based on body weight, age, and renal function. Most physicians obtain a serum digoxin concentration (SDC) once steady state is achieved (2 to 3 weeks), as a trough level drawn 6 hours or more after oral dosing. The SDC need not be repeated on a regular basis but should be determined in the setting of worsened renal function, signs or symptoms of digitalis toxicity, or the addition or discontinuation of drugs known to alter the SDC, such as amiodarone, quinidine, spironolactone, and others. An inital report suggested digoxin use increased mortality in women with heart failure, but mortality was later shown to be related to SDC, not gender.[61]

The effects of digoxin on the resting electrocardiogram (ECG) are well described. Although digoxin toxicity is a clinical diagnosis, it typically manifests as either excitatory (supraventricular tachycardia with block or ventricular extrasystoles, tachycardia, or fibrillation) or suppressant rhythm disturbances (sinus bradycardia, sinoatrial or atrioventricular block).

Diuretics

There are no clinical trial data prospectively evaluating the overall impact of diuretic therapy on mortality in the heart failure patient population. Clearly, diuretics are useful and necessary adjuncts to medical therapy for congestive heart failure symptoms caused by sodium and water retention, but they do not maintain clinical stability when used as monotherapy. While diuretics promote renal sodium and water excretion, they activate the renin-angiotensin-aldosterone axis, potentiate hypotensive effects of ACE inhibitors, and may decrease cardiac output if overused, especially in patients with diastolic LVD. Generally, diuretics create electrolyte wasting and attributable side effects.[62-70] Diuretic prescriptions should generally be accompanied by a recommendation for a dietary sodium restriction of 2,000 to 3,000 mg/d for the typical patient with heart failure. Fluid restriction is best reserved for the patient with excessive oral fluid intake, symptomatic hyponatremia, or diuretic refractoriness.

Diuretics should be used for congestive symptoms or signs and titrated according to an estimated 'dry' weight, which is based on optimal filling pressures and symptoms, without exacerbating symptomatic hypotension. Underuse of diuretic therapy is common, but excessive diuresis-limiting ventricular preload may, in turn, limit the blood pressure tolerance to oral vasodilator titration. Appropriate use of diuretic therapy is a key element in heart failure pharmacology. Intensification of diuretic and/or vasodilator therapy may be accompanied by a modest elevation and plateau in blood urea nitrogen and serum creatinine concentration. While often troubling to physicians, this finding is typically 'physiologic' and not considered indicative of intrinsic or irreversible renal dysfunction.

Generally, the most potent and widely used diuretic agents for heart failure management are the loop of Henle-active agents.

Loop Diuretics

Drugs acting on the ascending limb of the renal medullary loop of Henle are effective agents for the treatment of heart failure (Table 11-9). They are actively secreted in the proximal renal tubule and, therefore, depend on glomerular filtration to reach their site of action. Each drug has a maximum fractional excretion of filtered sodium (FeNa) of 20% to 25%, reflecting increased potency when compared with an FeNa of only 5% to 10% for the thiazide group.

Diuretic efficacy depends on the peak serum concentration reaching the renal glomeruli. Heart failure can affect drug pharmacokinetics in several ways. Delayed sorption caused by gut edema from high central venous pressure can reduce the peak serum concentration. The volume of distribution is also variable in the setting of chronic heart failure. Further, relative hypotension or reduced cardiac output that produces a limitation in renal blood flow reduces the glomerular filtration rate (GFR).

Generally, the limitations of loop diuretics can be overcome by successively increasing the administered dose. For the patient with profound fluid overload, continuous infusion of a loop diuretic can result in a 'steady-state' diuresis,[71] along with a more predictable rate of electrolyte loss that requires replacement. Similarly, some evidence shows that bumetanide (Bumex®) has greater efficacy than furosemide (Lasix®) in the setting of markedly reduced glomerular filtration, probably caused by proximal tubular filtration when secretion is limited. A continuous infusion of furosemide (0.05 to 0.1 mg/kg/h) or bumetanide (0.5 to 2 mg/h) has been shown to augment diuresis without excessive electrolyte loss. Inadequate diuresis and failure to assess the efficacy of oral diuretic administration before hospital discharge are common management errors leading to rapid symptomatic relapse and readmission.

With rapid IV administration of high-dose loop diuretics, hearing loss to the point of deafness can result from middle-ear toxicity. Skin reactions, from photosensitivity to rashes, are not uncommon, and hypersensitivity reactions can also manifest as interstitial nephritis. High doses of loop diuretics can worsen hyperglycemia and carbohydrate intolerance. Perhaps the most unpleasant and perplexing side effects of loop diuretics for patients with chronic heart failure are hyperuricemia and gout, which are caused by uric acid reabsorption.

Thiazide Diuretics

Thiazide diuretics inhibit sodium reabsorption in the distal renal tubule. They are generally not useful as diuretic monotherapy in heart failure and are ineffective when the GFR falls below 30 mL/min. In addition, to

Table 11-9: Commonly Used Diuretic Agents

Agent	Form	Dose Range	Maximum Daily Total Dose
Loop diuretics			
furosemide (Lasix®)	IV	10-200 mg	200 mg
	PO	20-200 mg q.d.-b.i.d.	400 mg
bumetanide (Bumex®)	IV	0.5-2 mg	10 mg
	PO	1.0-4 mg q.d.-b.i.d.	10 mg
torsemide (Demadex®)	IV	10-200 mg	200 mg
	PO	10-200 mg q.d.	200 mg
ethacrynic acid (Edecrin®)	Not available in United States		
Thiazide diuretics			
chlorothiazide (Diuril®)	IV	500-1,000 mg q.d.-b.i.d.	2,000 mg
	PO	500-1,000 mg q.d.-b.i.d.	2,000 mg

Duration of Action	Comment
	Generally effective diuretic mono-therapy in heart failure. Inhibit active NaCl transport in medullary ascending limb of the loop of Henle. Potassium and magnesium loss may require replacement.
~2-4 h	↓ efficacy with CrCl <30.
~6-8 h	↓↓ absorption in systemic venous congestion.
~2-4 h	Retains efficacy when CrCl <30 or if azotemia is present.
~6-8 h	↓ absorption with systemic venous congestion.
~3-6 h	Near 100% oral bioavailability.
~6-12 h	
	Only loop diuretic without a sulfhy-dryl group for sulfa-allergic patients.
	Generally not effective as monotherapy in moderate to severe heart failure. Act on distal convoluted tubule and cortical ascending limb of the loop of Henle.
~2-4 h	Used as adjunct to potentiate loop diuretic efficacy when higher doses of the former are required, with marked increase in electrolyte loss.
~6-8 h	

(continued on next page)

Table 11-9: Commonly Used Diuretic Agents
(continued)

Agent	Form	Dose Range	Maximum Daily Total Dose
Thiazide diuretics *(continued)*			
hydrochlorothiazide (HydroDIURIL®, Oretic®)	PO	25-50 mg q.d.	200 mg
metolazone (Mykrox®, Zaroxolyn®)	PO	2.5-5.0 mg b.i.d.	10 mg
Potassium-sparing diuretics			
amiloride (Midamor®)	PO	5-20 mg q.d.	20 mg
triamterene (Dyrenium®)	PO	100 mg b.i.d	200 mg
spironolactone (Aldactone®)	PO	12.5-200 mg q.d. in divided doses	200 mg
Eplerenone (Inspra®)	PO	25-50 mg q.d.	100 mg daily in divided doses (HTN), 50 mg daily (HF following MI)

PO = oral; IV = intravenous; q.d. = daily
b.i.d. = twice daily; q.o.d. = alternating days
CrCl = creatinine clearance
NYHA = New York Heart Association

Duration of Action	Comment
~6-12 h	
~8-24 h	
	Generally not used as monotherapy in heart failure. Helpful in patients with potassium wasting on loop diuretics. Frequent monitoring for hyperkalemia is advisable.
18-24 h	
~8 h	Do not combine with furosemide (prevents furosemide secretion).
8-24 h	Recommended for use in NYHA Class III-IV HF at 12.5-25 mg q.d. or q.o.d. for neurohormonal modulation. Monitor serum potassium closely.
	Subject to cytochrome P450 metabolism and drug interactions. Contraindicated if CrCl<30 ml/min in HF, or if CrCl <50 mL/min in HTN
	MI=myocardial infarction HTN=hypertension HF=heart failure

achieve a volume diuresis equivalent to that with loop diuretics, thiazides produce greater potassium wasting. Metolazone (Mykrox®, Zaroxolyn®) is particularly potent in this regard, acting in concert on proximal and distal tubules. Thiazide diuretics share most of the side effects seen with loop diuretics, although an association with pancreatitis appears be unique to this drug category.

Thiazide diuretics can be used in combination with loop diuretics to augment natriuresis when the dose of the loop diuretic is near maximum.[72-76] Diuretic resistance is partly related to chronic loop diuretic administration, typically at escalating doses. Chronic exposure results in progressive hypertrophy of distal renal tubular endothelial cells, which reabsorb sodium more avidly. By combining a thiazide diuretic with a loop-active drug, this compensatory hypertrophy can be overridden. The cost, however, is significant electrolyte loss. Therefore, the combination should primarily be used for patients refractory to high-dose loop diuretics.

Potassium-sparing Diuretics

Potassium (K)-sparing diuretics are used infrequently for direct diuretic activity, which is mild. Several are formulated in combination with thiazides for the treatment of hypertension, but they are generally not useful in heart failure. For patients with excessive potassium loss on loop diuretics, coincident administration of these agents can be helpful.

The use of spironolactone (Aldactone®) at a low dose (12.5 to 25 mg/d) as a systemic neurohormonal (aldosterone) antagonist for New York Heart Association (NYHA) Class III and IV patients is reviewed earlier in this chapter. When spironolactone is used, even in small doses, care must be taken to monitor frequently for the development of hyperkalemia, particularly in patients with preexisting renal insufficiency (serum creatinine >2.4 mg/dL) or with renal tubular acidosis. Between 10% and 15% of patients on chronic spironolactone therapy develop painful gynecomastia, which resolves upon discontinuation.

Alternative or Additional Vasodilator Therapy

Patients with chronic heart failure often benefit from the addition of a vasodilator to standard medical therapy, particularly when blood pressure remains relatively preserved.[22,23] Other patients may be unable to tolerate ACE inhibition because of rash, intractable cough, or angioedema.

Venous and arterial vasodilator therapy influences cardiac output and ventricular filling pressures in a failing ventricle with reduced contractility. Arterial vasodilation increases cardiac output while reducing LV end-diastolic pressure; venodilation reduces filling pressures (symptoms) with minimal effect on cardiac output. ACE inhibitor therapy as a neurohormonal antagonist with vasodilatory activity derived from positive results in early comparative vasodilator trials. ACE inhibitors and ARBs are compared earlier in this chapter.

Hydralazine and Isosorbide Dinitrate

The Vasodilator Heart Failure Trial (V-HeFT)[77] was the first randomized, placebo-controlled trial to assess the effect of the combination of a direct arterial vasodilator (hydralazine hydrochloride [Hz]) and a venous vasodilator (isosorbide dinitrate [ISDN]) with an α-1 antagonist (prazosin [Minipress®]) on survival in patients with heart failure. At the time, the trial was considered large, with 642 patients predominantly in NYHA Classes III and IV. The Hz plus ISDN combination (hydralazine 300 mg/day and isosorbide dinitrate 160 mg/day) had a significantly favorable effect on survival compared with placebo or prazosin (20 mg/day). Mortality was reduced by 23% with Hz plus ISDN, while the α-blocker provided no advantage over placebo, with a 1-year mortality risk of approximately 20%.

V-HeFT II[78] compared the relative efficacy of Hz plus ISDN to that of enalapril (Vasotec®) in reducing mortality in 804 men with chronic heart failure and an LVEF <0.45. The target doses were: hydralazine 75 mg q.i.d., isosorbide dinitrate 40 q.i.d. (with a 10-hour drug-free interval at night), and enalapril 10 mg b.i.d. Two-year mortality was lower in the enalapril group (18% vs 25%, P=0.016), and this difference persisted throughout the 5-year follow-up period. The Hz plus ISDN arm of V-HeFT II confirmed the findings of V-HeFT, with an annual mortality risk of 13% on active therapy. Interestingly, while enalapril therapy improved survival to a greater degree (9% annually), the Hz plus ISDN group had greater improvements in exercise capacity and LVEF.

For patients with significant renal insufficiency precluding the use of ACE inhibitors or ARBs,[79] the combination of Hz plus ISDN is an effective alternative therapy because it tends to increase renal cortical blood flow. While the hemodynamic effects of hydralazine in heart failure have been extensively studied, hydralazine has not been evaluated as monotherapy in heart failure mortality trials. Administration yields a reduction in systemic and pulmonary vascular resistance that augments stroke volume and cardiac output. The 5% to 10% reduction in mean arterial pressure results from a greater reduction in diastolic vs systolic pressure. While vasodilation is hemodynamically advantageous, it produces a reflex tachycardia that stimulates the sympathetic nervous system and increases renin activity in plasma (presumably as a result of increased secretion of renin by the renal juxtaglomerular cells in response to reflex sympathetic discharge). Heightened renin-angiotensin-aldosterone and sympathetic nervous system tone are considered disadvantageous in chronic heart failure. The side effect and dosing profiles of hydralazine are listed in Table 11-10.

Similarly, the independent effect of nitrates on survival in chronic heart failure is unknown. Isosorbide dinitrate was the active agent responsible for the improvement in exercise tolerance found in the V-HeFT trials. However, its use does not result in a sustained increase in systemic catecholamines. These agents facilitate improvement in peripheral vasodilator capacity, and nitrate administration helps restore endothelial endogenous nitric oxide synthase function by serving as a source of nitric oxide. Nitrates are useful as adjunctive therapy for symptomatic relief in patients with heart failure caused by underlying ischemic heart disease, those with subendocardial ischemia caused by increased wall stress, and those with moderate pulmonary hypertension. Nitrates reduce the effective mitral regurgitant orifice area and seem to improve ventricular diastolic function as well. Avoidance of pharmacodynamic tolerance can be easily accomplished by scheduling nitrate-free intervals.[80,81] The administration of hydralazine in combination with isosorbide dinitrate also seems to minimize the development of nitrate tolerance. Nitrate formulations are available in sustained-release forms, as well as in the mononitrate formulation, which is a primary metabolite of isosorbide dinitrate. The side effect profile of isosorbide can be found in Table 11-11.

A new, fixed-dose combination of 20 mg of isosorbide dinitrate and 37.5 mg of hydralazine hydrochloride (BiDil®) has been approved by the FDA for the treatment of heart failure as an adjunct to standard therapy in self-identified black patients, based on the results of the African-American Heart Failure Trial (A-HeFT).[81-85] Most of the patients in this trial had moderate to severe heart failure and were on baseline therapy, including a loop diuretic, an ACE inhibitor or an ARB, and a β-blocker. Many also were taking digoxin and/or an aldosterone antagonist. Compared with placebo, the addition of the combination hydralazine 225 mg/day and isosorbide dinitrate 120 mg/day was shown to improve survival by 43%, to reduce first heart failure hospitalizations by 39%, and to significantly improve patient-reported quality of life.[81] While the hydralazine/isosorbide combination was associated with a reduction in heart failure exacerbations (particularly severe exacerbations), it also significantly increased the side effects of headache and dizziness.

Table 11-10: Hydralazine*

Side Effect Profile

Common

- Headache, anorexia, vomiting, diarrhea, palpitations, tachycardia, angina pectoris

Less Frequent

- *Digestive:* constipation, paralytic ileus
- *Cardiovascular:* hypotension, paradoxical pressor response, edema
- *Respiratory:* dyspnea
- *Neurologic:* peripheral neuritis, evidenced by paresthesia, numbness, and tingling; dizziness; tremors; muscle cramps; psychotic reactions characterized by depression, disorientation, or anxiety
- *Genitourinary:* difficulty urinating
- *Hematologic:* blood dyscrasias, consisting of reduction in hemoglobin and red cell count, leukopenia, agranulocytosis, purpura, lymphadenopathy, splenomegaly

Calcium-channel Blockers

First-generation calcium-channel blockers (CCBs) are not recommended for use in heart failure because of systolic ventricular dysfunction caused by myocardial depressant (negative inotropic) effects.[22,23,86] Newer dihydropyridine CCB drugs, such as amlodipine (Norvasc®) and felodipine (Plendil®), have greater vasoselectivity (fewer myocardial depressant effects) and have been studied in heart failure populations.[87-90] They appear to have neutral effects on patient neurohormonal profile. However, their use has appeal for the treatment

Side Effect Profile (continued)
Less Frequent (continued)

- *Hypersensitivity:* rash, urticaria, pruritus, fever, arthralgia, eosinophilia, and, rarely, hepatitis
- *Other:* nasal congestion, flushing, lacrimation, conjunctivitis

Heart Failure Dosing

- *Available dosages:* 10-mg, 25-mg, 50-mg, and 100-mg tablets; 20 mg/mL injection
- *Dose interval:* t.i.d. to q.i.d.
- *Total daily dose range:* 40 to 300 mg
- *Peak effect:* 1 to 2 h
- *Half-life:* 3 to 7 h

* Hydralazine is subject to polymorphic acetylation; slow acetylators generally have higher plasma levels of hydralazine and require or tolerate lower doses.

of angina or residual hypertension in patients on standard heart failure therapy who are intolerant of or who have strong contraindications to β-blockade. Patients with heart failure and preserved systolic function and/or LV hypertrophy may also derive symptomatic benefit from CCB therapy; however, no morbidity or mortality data exist to guide agent selection at this time. The peripheral vasodilatation induced by CCBs has the common side effect of peripheral edema, which may represent a confusing physical finding when evaluating signs of heart failure in individual patients.

Table 11-11: Isosorbide Dinitrate

Side Effect Profile

Common

- Headache may be severe and persistent

Less Common

- Cutaneous vasodilation with flushing

- Lightheadedness, dizziness, and weakness

- Hypotension may be accompanied by paradoxical bradycardia

- Additive effect to alcohol

- Marked additive and potentially fatal hypotension if combined with sildenafil (Viagra®)

Extremely Rare

- Methemoglobinemia

- Allergic reaction

Heart Failure Dosing

- *Available dosages:* 5-mg, 10-mg, 20-mg, 30-mg, and 40-mg tablets; 40-mg sustained-release capsules and tablets

- *Dose interval:* b.i.d. to q.i.d. (t.i.d. typical with 8 or more hours of nitrate-free interval)

- *Daily dose:* 30 to 480 mg

- *Average bioavailability:* approximately 25%

V-HeFT III examined the effects of felodipine on exercise capacity and survival in chronic heart failure as additive therapy to ACE inhibitors, digoxin, and diuretics. Felodipine treatment had no effect on mortality in this population, although there was a worrying trend toward an adverse outcome as the study progressed. There was also no benefit observed in exercise tolerance from active CCB therapy.

Amlodipine was evaluated in the Prospective Randomized Amlodipine Survival Evaluation (PRAISE) trials,[84,85] which added amlodipine or placebo to background heart failure therapy of an ACE inhibitor, digoxin, and diuretics. Although, overall, the trial demonstrated a neutral effect on survival, a retrospective subset analysis detected a significant improvement in survival in nonischemic heart failure patients. PRAISE-2 was conducted to further assess and validate this possibility in a population of patients with nonischemic cardiomyopathy and symptomatic heart failure. When evaluated prospectively, there was no survival advantage (or disadvantage) attributable to amlodipine administration in this population.

References

1.   Consensus recommendations for the management of chronic heart failure. On behalf of the membership of the advisory council to improve outcomes nationwide in heart failure. *Am J Cardiol* 1999;83:1A-38A.

2.   Eichhorn EJ, Bristow MR: Medical therapy can improve the biological properties of the chronically failing heart. A new treatment era of heart failure. *Circulation* 1996;94:2285-2296.

3.   Katz AM. In: Hosenpud JD, Greenberg BH: *Congestive Heart Failure*, 2nd ed. Philadelphia, Lippincott, Williams and Wilkins, 2000, pp 3-8.

4.   Bristow MR, Ginsburg R, Umans V, et al: β_1 and β_2-adrenergic subpopulations in nonfailing and failing human ventricular myocardium: coupling of both receptor subtypes to muscle contraction and selective β_1-receptor down regulation in heart failure. *Circ Res* 1989;59:297-309.

5.   Waagstein F, Hjalmarson A, Varnauskas E, et al: Effect of chronic β-adrenergic receptor blockades in congestive cardiomyopathy. *Br Heart J* 1975;37:1022-1036.

6.   Swedberg K, Hjalmarson A, Waagstein F, et al: Prolongation of survival in congestive cardiomyopathy by β-receptor blockade. *Lancet* 1979;1:1374-1376.

7.   Chadda K, Goldstein S, Byington R, et al: Effect of propranolol after acute myocardial infarction in patients with congestive heart failure. *Circulation* 1986;73:503-510.

8.   Fisher ML, Gottlieb SS, Plotnick GD, et al: Beneficial effects of metoprolol in heart failure associated with coronary artery disease: a randomized trial. *J Am Coll Cardiol* 1994;23:943-950.

9.   Eichhorn EJ, Heesch CM, Barnett JH, et al: Effect of metoprolol on myocardial function and energetics in patients with non-ischemic dilated cardiomyopathy: a randomized, double-blind, placebo-controlled study. *J Am Coll Cardiol* 1994;24:1310-1320.

10.   Hall SA, Cigarroa CG, Marcoux L, et al: Time course of improvement in left ventricular function, mass and geometry in patients with congestive heart failure treated with β-adrenergic blockade. *J Am Coll Cardiol* 1995;25:1154-1161.

11.   Olsen SL, Gilbert EM, Renlund DG, et al: Carvedilol improves left ventricular function and symptoms in chronic heart failure: a double-blind randomized study. *J Am Coll Cardiol* 1995;25:1225-1231.

12.   Waagstein F, Bristow MR, Swedburg K, et al: Beneficial effects of metoprolol in idiopathic dilated cardiomyopathy. *Lancet* 1993;342:1441-1446.

13.   A randomized trial of β-blockade in heart failure. The cardiac insufficiency bisoprolol study (CIBIS). CIBIS Investigators and Committee. *Circulation* 1994;90:1765-1773.

14.   Packer M, Bristow MR, Cohn JN, et al: The effect of carvedilol on morbidity and mortality in patients with chronic heart failure. U.S. Carvedilol Heart Failure Study Group. *N Engl J Med* 1996;334:1349-1355.

15.   The Cardiac Insufficiency Bisoprolol Study II (CIBIS-II): a randomised trial. *Lancet* 1999;353:9-13.

16.   Effect of metoprolol CR/XL in chronic heart failure: Metoprolol CR/XL Randomised Intervention Trial in Congestive Heart Failure (MERIT-HF). *Lancet* 1999;353:2001-2007.

17.   Talwar KK, Bhargava B, Upasani PT, et al: Hemodynamic prediction of early intolerance and long-term effects of propranolol in dilated cardiomyopathy. *J Card Fail* 1996;2:273-277.

18. Haber HL, Simek CL, Gimple LW, et al: Why do patients with congestive heart failure tolerate the initiation of β-blocker therapy? *Circulation* 1993;88:1610-1619.

19. A trial of the beta-blocker bucindolol in patients with advanced chronic heart failure. *N Engl J Med* 2001;344:1659-1667.

20. Packer M, Coats AJ, Fowler MB, et al: Effect of carvedilol on survival in severe chronic heart failure: results of the carvedilol prospective randomized cumulative survival (COPERNICUS) study. *N Engl J Med* 2001;344:1651-1658.

21. Poole-Wilson PA, Swedberg K, Cleland JG, et al: Comparison of carvedilol and metoprolol on clinical outcomes in patients with chronic heart failure in the Carvedilol Or Metoprolol European Trial (COMET): randomised controlled trial. *Lancet* 2003;362:7-13.

22. Hunt SA, Abraham WT, Chin MH, et al: ACC/AHA 2005 Guideline Update for the Diagnosis and Management of Chronic Heart Failure in the Adult: a report of the American College of Cardiology/American Heart Association Task Force on Practice Guidelines (Writing Committee to Update the 2001 Guidelines for the Evaluation and Management of Heart Failure): developed in collaboration with the American College of Chest Physicians and the International Society for Heart and Lung Transplantation: endorsed by the Heart Rhythm Society. *Circulation* 2005;112:e154-235.

23. Heart Failure Society of America. HFSA 2006 Comprehensive Heart Failure Practice Guideline. *J Card Fail* 2006;12:e1-2. Full guideline available at http://www.heartfailureguideline.com.

24. Gattis WA, O'Connor CM, Gallup DS, et al: Predischarge initiation of carvedilol in patients hospitalized for decompensated heart failure: results of the Initiation Management Predischarge: Process for Assessment of Carvedilol Therapy in Heart Failure (IMPACT-HF) trial. *J Am Coll Cardiol* 2004;43:1534-1541.

25. Randomised, placebo-controlled trial of carvedilol in patients with congestive heart failure due to ischaemic heart disease. Australia/New Zealand Heart Failure Research Collaborative Group. *Lancet* 1997;349:375-380.

26. Waagstein F, Caidahl K, Wallentin I, et al: Long-term β-blockade in dilated cardiomyopathy. Effects of short- and long-term metoprolol treatment followed by withdrawal and readministration of metoprolol. *Circulation* 1989;80:551-563.

27.   Peng JF, Gurantz D, Cowling RT, et al: TNF-α alters Ang II-medicated cardiac fibroblast function in favor of fibrosis. *J Cardiol Failure* 2000;6:2-21.

28.   Farhy RD, Ho K, Carretero OA, et al: Kinins mediate the antiproliferative effect of ramipril in rat carotid artery. *Biochem Biophys Res Commun* 1992;182:283-288.

29.   Alderman MH, Madhavan SH, Ooi WL, et al: Association of the renin-sodium profile with the risk of myocardial infarction in patients with hypertension. *N Engl J Med* 1991;324:1098-1104.

30.   Yusuf S, Pepine CJ, Garces C, et al: Effect of enalapril on myocardial infarction and unstable angina in patients with low ejection fractions. *Lancet* 1992;340:1173-1178.

31.   Pfeffer MA, Braunwald E, Moyé LA, et al: Effect of captopril on mortality and morbidity in patients with left ventricular dysfunction after myocardial infarction. Results of the survival and ventricular enlargement trial. The SAVE Investigators. *N Engl J Med* 1992;327:669-677.

32.   Yusuf S, Sleight P, Pogue J, et al: Effects of an angiotensin-converting-enzyme inhibitor, ramipril, on cardiovascular events in high-risk patients. *N Engl J Med* 2000;342:145-153.

33.   Ambrosioni E, Borghi C, Magnani B: The effect of the angiotensin-converting-enzyme inhibitor zofenopril on mortality and morbidity after anterior myocardial infarction. The Survival of Myocardial Infarction Long-Term Evaluation (SMILE) Study Investigators. *N Engl J Med* 1995;332:80-85.

34.   Franzosi MG, Santoro E, Zuanetti G, et al: Indications for ACE inhibitors in the early treatment of acute myocardial infarction: systematic overview of individual data from 100,000 patients in randomized trials. *Circulation* 1998;97:2202-2212.

35.   Flather MD, Yusuf S, Kober L, et al: Long-term ACE-inhibitor therapy in patients with heart failure or left-ventricular dysfunction: a systematic overview of data from individual patients. ACE-Inhibitor Myocardial Infarction Collaborative Group. *Lancet* 2000;355:1575-1581.

36.   Effect of ramipril on mortality and morbidity of survivors of acute myocardial infarction with evidence of heart failure. The Acute Infarction Ramipril Efficacy (AIRE) Study Investigators. *Lancet* 1993;342:821-828.

37.   Yusuf S, Pitt B, Davis CE, et al: Effect of enalapril on mortality and the development of heart failure in asymptomatic patients

with reduced left ventricular ejection fractions. *N Engl J Med* 1992;327:685-691.

38. Effect of enalapril on survival in patients with reduced left ventricular ejection fractions and congestive heart failure. The SOLVD Investigators. *N Engl J Med* 1991;325:293-302.

39. Greenberg B, Quinones MA, Koilpillai C, et al: Effects of long-term enalapril therapy on cardiac structure and function in patients with left ventricular dysfunction. Results of the SOLVD echocardiography substudy. *Circulation* 1995;91:2573-2581.

40. Effects of enalapril on mortality in severe congestive heart failure. Results of the Cooperative North Scandinavian Enalapril Survival Study (CONSENSUS). The CONSENSUS Trial Study Group. *N Engl J Med* 1987;316:1429-1435.

41. Pitt B, Chang P, Timmermans PB: Angiotensin II receptor antagonists in heart failure: rationale and design of the evaluation of losartan in the elderly (ELITE) trial. *Cardiovasc Drugs Ther* 1995,9:693-700.

42. Goodfriend TL, Elliot ME, Catt KJ: Angiotensin receptors and their antagonists. *N Engl J Med* 1996;334:1649-1654.

43. Cheng CP, Onishi K, Ohte N, et al: Functional effects of endogenous bradykinin in congestive heart failure. *J Am Coll Cardiol* 1998;31:1679-1686.

44. Oudit GY, Crackower MA, Backx PH, et al: The role of ACE2 in cardiovascular physiology. *Trends Cardiovasc Med* 2003;13:93-101.

45. Ishiyama Y, Gallager PE, Averill DB, et al: Upregulation of angiotensin-converting enzyme 2 after myocardial infarction by blockade of angiotensin II receptors. *Hypertension* 2004;43:970-976.

46. Pitt B, Poole-Wilson PA, Segal R, et al: Effect of losartan compared with captopril on mortality in patients with symptomatic heart failure: randomized trial—the Losartan Heart Failure Survival Study ELITE II. *Lancet* 2000;355:1582-1587.

47. Pitt B, Segal R, Martinez FA, et al: Randomised trial of losartan versus captopril in patients over 65 with heart failure (Evaluation of Losartan in the Elderly Study, ELITE). *Lancet* 1997;349:747-752.

48. Maggioni AP, Anand I, Gottlieb SO, et al: Effects of valsartan on morbidity and mortality in patients with heart failure not re-

ceiving angiotensin-converting enzyme inhibitors. *J Am Coll Cardiol* 2002;40:1414-1421.

49. Granger CB, McMurray JJ, Yusuf S, et al: Effects of candesartan in patients with chronic heart failure and reduced left-ventricular systolic function intolerant to angiotensin-converting-enzyme inhibitors: The CHARM-Alternative Trial. *Lancet* 2003;362:772-776.

50. McMurray JJ, Ostergren J, Swedberg K, et al: Effects of candesartan in patients with chronic heart failure and reduced left-ventricular systolic function taking angiotensin-converting-enzyme inhibitors: the CHARM-Added trial. *Lancet* 2003;362:767-771.

51. McKelvie RS, Yusuf S, Pericak D, et al: Comparison of candesartan, enalapril, and their combination in congestive heart failure: randomized evaluation of strategies for left ventricular dysfunction (RESOLVD) pilot study. The RESOLVD Pilot Study Investigators. *Circulation* 1999;100:1056-1064.

52. Yusuf S, Pfeffer MA, Swedberg K, et al: Effects of candesartan in patients with chronic heart failure and preserved left-ventricular ejection fraction: the CHARM-Preserved trial. *Lancet* 2003;362:777-781.

53. Borghi C, Boschi S, Ambrosioni E, et al: Evidence of a partial escape of renin-angiotensin-aldosterone blockade in patients with acute myocardial infarction treated with ACE inhibitors. *J Clin Pharmacol* 1993;33:40-45.

54. Brilla CG, Rupp H, Funck R, et al: The renin-angiotensin-aldosterone system and myocardial collagen matrix remodelling in congestive heart failure. *Eur Heart J* 1995;16:107-109.

55. Weber KT: Extracellular matrix remodeling in heart failure: a role for de novo angiotensin II generation. *Circulation* 1997;96:4065-4082.

56. The effect of digoxin on mortality and morbidity in patients with heart failure. The Digitalis Investigation Group. *N Engl J Med* 1997;336:525-533.

57. Uretsky BF, Young JB, Shahidi FE, et al: Randomized study assessing the effect of digoxin withdrawal in patients with mild to moderate chronic congestive heart failure: results of the PROVED trial. PROVED Investigative Group. *J Am Coll Cardiol* 1993;22:955-962.

58. Packer M, Gheorghiade M, Young JB, et al: Withdrawal of digoxin from patients with chronic heart failure treated with an-

giotensin-converting enzyme inhibitors. RADIANCE Study. *N Engl J Med* 1993;329:1-7.

59. Gheorghiade M, Ferguson D: Digoxin. A neurohormonal modulator in heart failure? *Circulation* 1991;84:2181-2186.

60. Gheorghiade M, Hall VB, Jacobsen G, et al: Effects of increasing maintenance dose of digoxin on left ventricular function and neurohormones in patients with chronic heart failure treated with diuretics and angiotensin-converting enzyme inhibitors. *Circulation* 1995;92:1801-1807.

61. Adams KF Jr, Patterson JH, Gattis WA, et al: Relationship of serum digoxin concentration to mortality and morbidity in women in the digitalis investigation group trial: a retrospective analysis. *J Am Coll Cardiol* 2005;46:497-504.

62. Brater DC: Diuretic therapy. *N Engl J Med* 1998;339: 387-395.

63. Cody RJ, Covit AB, Schaer GL, et al: Sodium and water balance in chronic congestive heart failure. *J Clin Invest* 1986;77: 1441-1452.

64. Cody RJ, Kubo SH, Pickworth KK: Diuretic treatment for the sodium retention of congestive heart failure. *Arch Intern Med* 1994;154:1905-1914.

65. Domanski M, Tian X, Haigney M, et al: Diuretic use, progressive heart failure, and death in patients in the DIG study. *J Card Fail* 2006;12:327-332.

66. Eshaghian S, Horwich TB, Fonarow GC: Relation of loop diuretic dose to mortality in advanced heart failure. *Am J Cardiol* 2006;97:1759-1764

67. Rude RK: Physiology of magnesium metabolism and the important role of magnesium in potassium deficiency. *Am J Cardiol* 1989;63:31G-34G.

68. Leier CV, Dei Cas L, Metra M: Clinical relevance and management of the major electrolyte abnormalities in congestive heart failure: hyponatremia, hypokalemia and hypomagnesemia. *Am Heart J* 1994:128:564-574.

69. Risler T, Schwab A, Kramer B, et al: Comparative pharmacokinetics and pharmacodynamics of loop diuretics in renal failure. *Cardiology* 1994;84(suppl 2):155-161.

70. Patterson JH, Adams KF Jr, Applefeld MM, et al: Oral torsemide in patients with chronic congestive heart failure: effects

on body weight, edema, and electrolyte excretion. Torsemide Investigators Group. *Pharmacotherapy* 1994;14:514-521.

71.   Aaser E, Gullestad L, Tollofsrud S, et al: Effect of bolus injection versus continuous infusion of furosemide on diuresis and neurohormonal activation in patients with severe congestive heart failure. *Scand J Clin Lab Invest* 1997;57:361-367.

72.   Sica DA, Deedwania P: Pharmacotherapy in congestive heart failure. Principles of combination diuretic therapy in congestive heart failure. *Congest Heart Fail* 1997;3:29-38.

73.   Sica DA, Gehr TW: Diuretic combinations in refractory oedema states: pharmacokinetic-pharmacodynamic relationships. *Clin Pharmacokinet* 1996;30:229-249.

74.   Dormans TP, Gerlad PG, Russell FG, et al: Combination diuretic therapy in severe congestive heart failure. *Drugs* 1998;55:165-172.

75.   Ellison DH: The physiologic basis of diuretic synergism: its role in treating diuretic resistance. *Ann Intern Med* 1991;114:886-894.

76.   Epstein M, Lepp BA, Hoffman DS, et al: Potentiation of furosemide by metolazone in refractory edema. *Curr Ther Res Clin Exp*1977;21:656-667.

77.   Cohn JN, Archibald DG, Ziesche S, et al: Effect of vasodilator therapy on mortality in chronic congestive heart failure. Results of a Veterans Administration Cooperative Study. *N Engl J Med* 1986;314:1547-1552.

78.   Cohn JN, Johnson G, Ziesche S, et al: A comparison of enalapril with hydralazine-isosorbide dinitrate in the treatment of chronic congestive heart failure. *N Engl J Med* 1991;325:303-310.

79.   Packer M, Lee WH, Medina N, et al: Functional renal insufficiency during long-term therapy with captopril and enalapril in severe chronic heart failure. *Ann Intern Med* 1987;106:346-354.

80.   Abrams J: Beneficial actions of nitrates in cardiovascular disease. *Am J Cardiol* 1996;77:31C-37C.

81.   Gogia H, Mehra A, Parikh S, et al: Prevention of tolerance to hemodynamic effects of nitrates with concomitant use of hydralazine in patients with chronic heart failure. *J Am Coll Cardiol* 1995;26:1575-1580.

82.   Taylor AL, Ziesche S, Yancy C, et al: Combination of isosorbide dinitrate and hydralazine in blacks with heart failure. *N Engl J Med* 2004;351:2049-2057.

83. Exner DV, Dries DL, Domanski MJ, et al: Lesser response to angiotensin-converting-enzyme inhibitor therapy in blacks as compared with white patients with left ventricular dysfunction. *N Engl J Med* 2001;344:1351-1357.

84. Dries DL, Exner DV, Gersh BJ, et al: Racial differences in the outcome of left ventricular dysfunction. *N Engl J Med* 1999; 340:609-616.

85. Wallace TW, Drazner MH: The impact of race on response to RAAS inhibition. *Curr Heart Failure Rep* 2005;2:72-77.

86. Yancy CW: Heart failure in African Americans: a cardiovascular enigma. *J Card Fail* 2000;6:183-186.

87. Cohn JN, Ziesche S, Smith R, et al: Effect of the calcium antagonist felodipine as supplementary vasodilator therapy in patients with chronic heart failure treated with enalapril: V-HeFT III. Vasodilator-Heart Failure Trial (V-HeFT) Study Group. *Circulation* 1997;96:856-863.

88. Tan LB, Murray RG, Littler WA: Felodipine in patients with chronic heart failure: discrepant haemodynamic and clinical effects. *Br Heart J* 1987;58:122-128.

89. Packer M, O'Connor CM, Ghali JK, et al: Effect of amlodipine on morbidity and mortality in severe chronic heart failure. Prospective Randomized Amlodipine Survival Evaluation Study Group. *N Engl J Med* 1996;335:1107-1114.

90. Cabell CH, Trichon BH, Velazquez EJ, et al: Importance of echocardiography in patients with severe nonischemic heart failure: the second Prospective Randomized Amlodipine Survival Evaluation (PRAISE-2) echocardiographic study. *Am Heart J* 2004;147:151-157.

Index

Valsartan in Heart Failure Trial (Val-HeFT) 79, 320, 321, 325, 344
valvular heart disease 265, 274
valvular insufficiency 247
vascular disease 171, 173, 223, 278
vascular dysfunction 271
vascular insufficiency 267
vasoconstriction 246, 294
vasodilation 295, 340, 343
vasodilator 241, 267, 339
Vasodilator Heart Failure Trial (V-HeFT) 339, 340
Vasotec® 74, 172, 174, 307, 315, 339
vegetables 13, 14, 51, 54, 55
ventricular arrhythmias 78, 143, 148, 183, 187
ventricular dysfunction 265, 274, 276, 278, 280, 282, 284
ventricular fibrillation 182
ventricular impairment 270
ventricular tachycardia 141
verapamil (Calan®, Covera-HS®, Isoptin®, Verelan®) 85, 96, 179, 180, 224
Verelan® 179, 224

very low-density lipoprotein (VLDL) 15, 56, 88, 89, 92, 199
very low-density lipoprotein cholesterol (VLDL-C) 14
Veterans Affairs High-Density Lipoprotein Cholesterol Intervention Trial (VA-HIT) 200
Visken® 81
vitamin B12 220, 221, 223
vitamin B6 220, 221, 223
vitamin C 55, 221
Vitamin E 220
vitamin E 55, 221
volleyball 57
volume load 248, 253
volume overload 242, 252, 263, 276, 277, 292, 298
vomiting 342

W

waist circumference 11, 27, 32, 36, 39, 41, 42
walking 12, 56, 57
wall stress 246, 247, 252, 256, 291
warfarin (Coumadin®) 98, 155, 185
Warfarin Reinfarction Study (WARIS) 155
water retention 246, 253, 254, 272, 291, 326, 331

weight control 54
weight gain 12, 62, 80, 266, 301
weight loss 11, 12, 46-48, 50, 62, 266
weight management 223
weight reduction 48, 49, 51, 226
Welchol® 98
West of Scotland Coronary Prevention Study (WOSCOP 93, 204
wheezes 275, 277
whole grains 14, 54, 55
Women's Ischemic Syndrome Evaluation (WISE) study 233
World Health Organization (WHO) 21, 33-36, 39, 40, 66, 71, 99

World Health Organization (WHO) *(continued)*
Monitoring Trends and Determinants of Cardiovascular Disease (MONICA) 180

X

Xenical® 50

Z

Zaroxolyn® 336, 338
Zebeta® 80, 293, 294
Zestril® 174, 315
Zetia® 97, 213
Zocor® 93, 202
zofenopril 172
Zyban® 61, 223

NOTES